LIVE A
BEAUTIFUL
LIFE

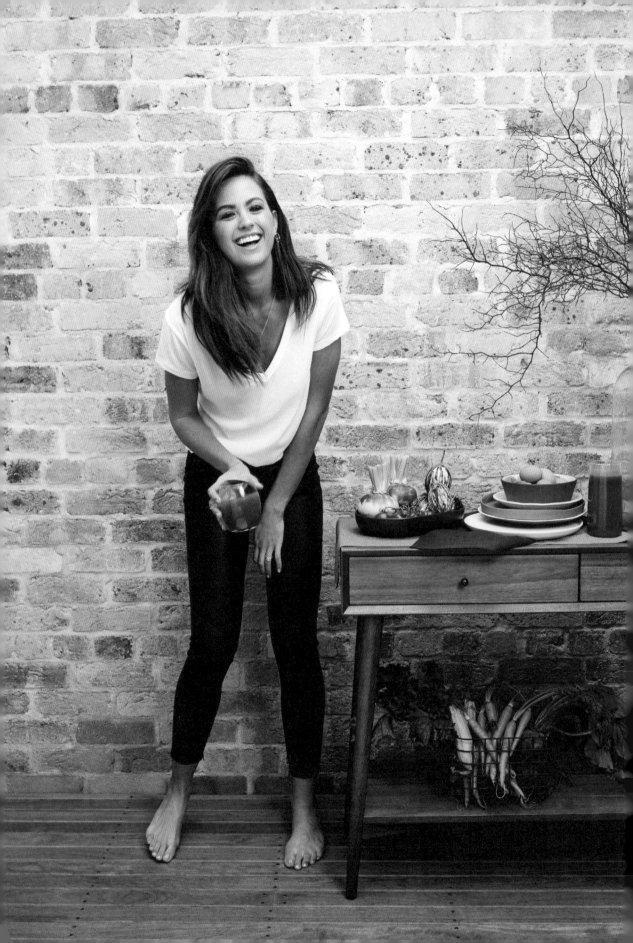

LIVE A
BEAUTIFUL
LIFE

Jesinta Campbell

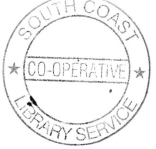

hachette
AUSTRALIA

Contents

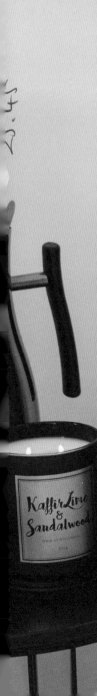

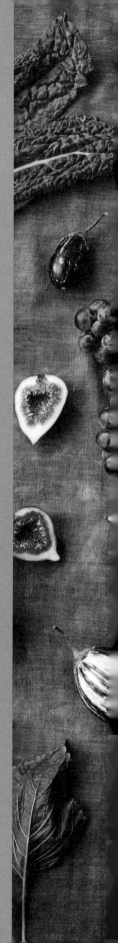

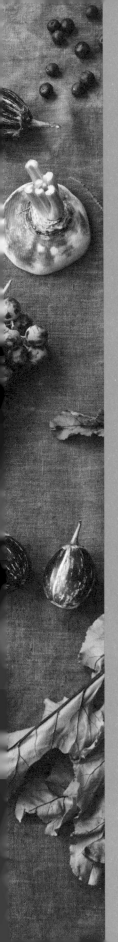

Dinner 178

Big Dreams 214

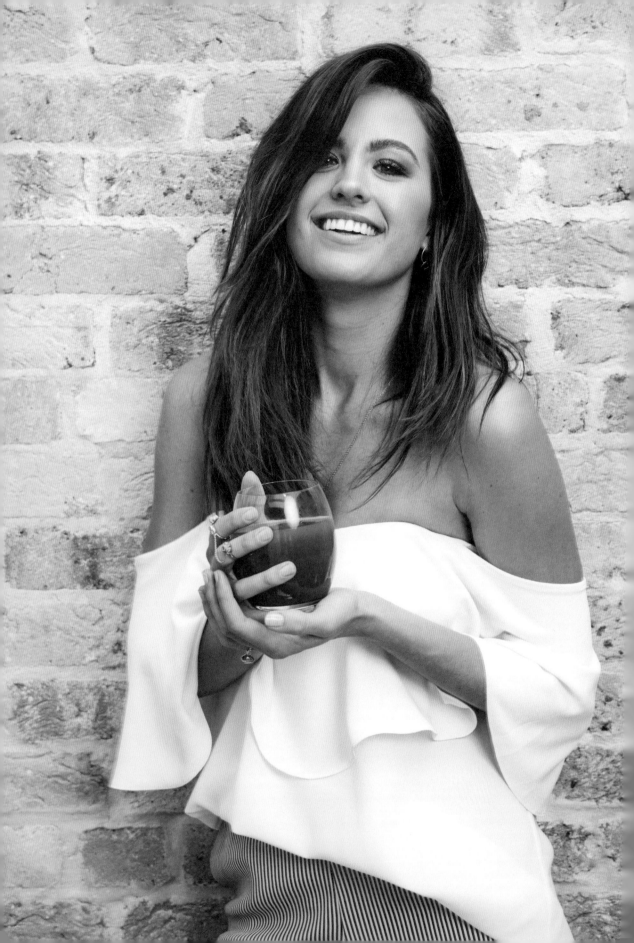

Welcome

Firstly, thank you. Thank you for allowing me to be a part of your journey. And congratulations on taking a step towards a healthier, fitter, better version of YOU!

I was inspired to put together this book because I am passionate about living a healthy, active life and often get asked questions about my workouts, the food I eat, my beauty routine and what motivates me. I don't claim to be an expert in nutrition, fitness, beauty or motivation; however, I have learnt through my own personal experiences what makes me happy and what works for me.

My goal is that this book will inspire you to be the best version of you that you can possibly be. Everyone is different, our experiences and stories shape who we are, and it's these differences that make you unique.

I hope you enjoy this little project that I've been working on especially for you. It has been an amazing experience writing this book. A lot of love and care has gone into creating something that I hope you will gain a lot from. Every workout, recipe, quote and picture was chosen with you in mind.

Lots of love,

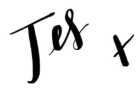

Jes x

Health & Wellness

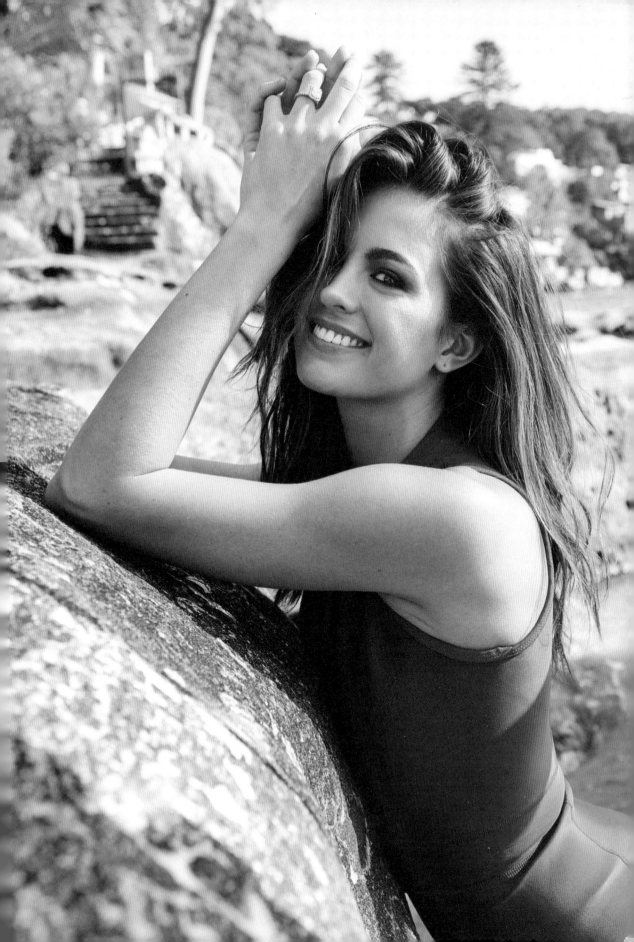

I HAVE ALWAYS BEEN an advocate of living an active, healthy lifestyle and the older I get the more I appreciate my health.

For me, being healthy is like a puzzle, with many different pieces that need to come together in order to create the full picture. Being healthy means keeping fit, eating right, getting enough sleep, and of course looking after my mind and mental wellbeing. It is about finding the right balance for you and your body and maintaining it.

The importance of health is definitely something that was instilled in me from a young age. I grew up in a household where we were encouraged to express ourselves, communicate, work through our challenges and not bottle up our emotions. The importance of being in touch with your emotions and knowing how to work through difficult situations is vital to minimise stress in your life. Family was always a safe place for us to talk and work through things.

We didn't have packaged food in the pantry or soft drink in the fridge. If we wanted cookies or muffins for our lunch boxes, Mum and Dad would encourage us to bake them ourselves. This is where I learnt the importance of nutrition and eating food as close to its natural form as possible. To this day I still make as much as I can from scratch, it doesn't take much extra effort and it means I know exactly what is in my food and what I am putting into my body. I love nothing more than doing a massive grocery shop or heading to the local farmers' markets on a Sunday to stock up my kitchen with lots and lots of vegetables and fruit, so that I have a great range of fresh produce to work with. I love being able to make my own fresh juices and smoothies, and instead of reaching for a packet of chips when the afternoon munchies kick in, I snack on crisp veggie sticks.

When I was growing up, Mum and Dad didn't place any importance on how my sister and I looked, our body weight or how or when we exercised. We were brought up on acreage so we were always encouraged to go outside and play instead of being indoors. We didn't watch much television; hardly any at all, actually, and never played computer games. Mum would go running a couple of times a week around the river with her friends and when I was thirteen I decided that I wanted to join in. At that stage in my life it was something fun and social to do.

Looking back I think this natural progression into exercise is why I still love training to this day. For me, it was never a chore and my parents were very conscious to make sure that exercise was never about weight loss or how my body looked – the focus was on how it made me feel and the sense of achievement I got when I completed something I had set out to do.

Too often, especially for women, we make exercise about losing weight. Yes, getting toned and looking fit is a great by-product of exercise; however, I challenge you to change your mindset around why you workout. For me, exercise is a stress reliever, something that challenges me and something I actually enjoy. I love to exercise. Moving my limbs, the sweat on my forehead, the thirst, the feeling of blood pumping around my body, the challenge, and the pain, then the exhilaration. The biggest thing I have learnt about exercise is that it shouldn't be about how it makes you look, but rather about how it makes you FEEL!

Life has presented me with some extremely challenging times over the past couple of years. A plethora of pressures present themselves alongside my career; living a life in the public eye since I was thrust into the spotlight aged eighteen after winning Miss Universe Australia has proven difficult at times. What I wear, what I do, where I go, who I hang out with and who I date are scrawled all over the pages of magazines, gossip columns and social media across the country.

Over the years there have been just as many ups as there have been downs. Recently, my fiancé's battle with mental illness was made public after he took time-out from playing football as his team approached the finals. At the time, I could go to the gym, put my music in and train, and for that hour nothing else occupied my mind other than what was happening in the present moment. I learnt that looking after my health means I'm in the best shape to take on the challenges in life.

My top tips for a healthy life

A HEALTHY BODY MEANS a healthy mind; I do not believe you can have one without the other! Too often we think healthy is just about the exercise we do, or the food we eat. I can't talk about fitness without talking about health and nutrition and vice versa. If you want to achieve optimum fitness and health, there are many pieces of the puzzle that you need to put together. This includes rest, relaxation, a balanced diet and regular exercise. So here are my top tips for a healthy life:

1. Exercise regularly

Exercise is known to improve your overall wellbeing. Even a brisk walk in the fresh air can instantly lighten your mood. If I'm having a bad day or need to make an important decision, I will often go for a walk or light run. I find it brings me clarity and I end up in a better place than I was before I exercised.

Nothing beats the feeling of being fit and strong. Being able to walk up a steep set of stairs without puffing, the ability to run around with your dog in the park without getting exhausted, and fitting into your favourite pair of jeans are the simple things that feel really good when you are fit.

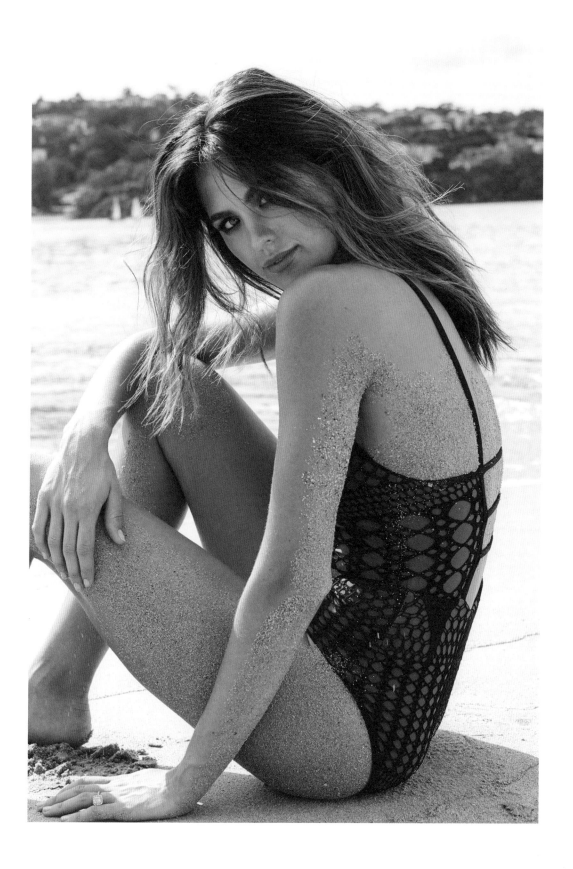

2. Eat clean, wholesome food

There is no such thing as a quick fix when it comes to your diet. What I've learnt is that balance is key. The trick with nutrition is to find out what works for you. Find where your body sits naturally and comfortably and aim to maintain that. Don't slave your life away to try to be something you're not. Food should be enjoyed and used as fuel for your body.

My general rule is Monday to Friday I eat wholesome, organic food. Saturday, I like to have a glass of wine, and on Sunday – Funday! – I indulge a little. I have a naughty sweet tooth so I like chocolate or something to satisfy it. A treat now and then keeps you sane and you don't feel like you are depriving yourself! I don't drink soft drink; I never have and would recommend that you cut that crap out of your diet ASAP!

I mainly eat fish and chicken during the week. Sometimes I crave red meat so I'll have that, but not very often. Vegetables are an absolute must, and if I feel like I haven't had enough in the day I'll make myself a big smoothie with 2–3 handfuls of spinach in it.

For snacks, I make up a batch of protein balls or I eat a variety of nuts, fruit or veggie sticks with a dip like guacamole.

Nutrition is a big part of the picture when it comes to your health and fitness. There is no point spending time working out then ruining it with bad food choices. Keep it clean during the week.

I don't believe in dieting, I believe in making healthy food choices every day. If I have a big swimsuit shoot or show coming up, I will cut out sugar and alcohol. But if I maintain good nutrition all year round, then it's easier to stay in shape and I always feel healthy. I also believe in not making healthy eating a chore – have fun experimenting in the kitchen, invite people over for dinner and always enjoy what you eat!

3. Hydrate

Hydration is so important for your body to function at its optimum. It sounds super simplistic but not enough people consume enough H_2O.

— —

Water

Approximately 60 per cent of our bodies are made up of water and the majority of us do not drink enough in order to stay well hydrated.

For me, water is the cure for everything. Before I take a painkiller for a headache, I make sure I drink one or two glasses of water and wait half an hour, because unless my headache is hormonal it's usually due to being dehydrated. Before I reach for the 4pm sugar hit, I'll hydrate as most of the time I am thirsty, not hungry! Water reduces my cravings and after a little bit I am no longer screaming for something sweet.

The biggest difference I notice when I drink lots of water is that my skin completely changes; it glows from the inside out.

And if I'm not wearing makeup or I'm on holidays, I only clean my face with warm water – no products are required to clean the skin or keep it healthy.

If you want to increase your consumption of water, here are my simple tricks. Drink a big glass of water as soon as you wake up. Buy yourself a nice glass or stainless steel bottle and take it with you EVERYWHERE you go. If it is sitting on your desk or in your handbag, you are more likely to drink it throughout the day. Squeeze a bit of lemon in it or add some chopped apple, berries and mint to give it a hint of flavour.

Watch your skin change, eyes become brighter and find greater focus simply by increasing your intake of water during the day. It is the top of my list of health priorities.

— —

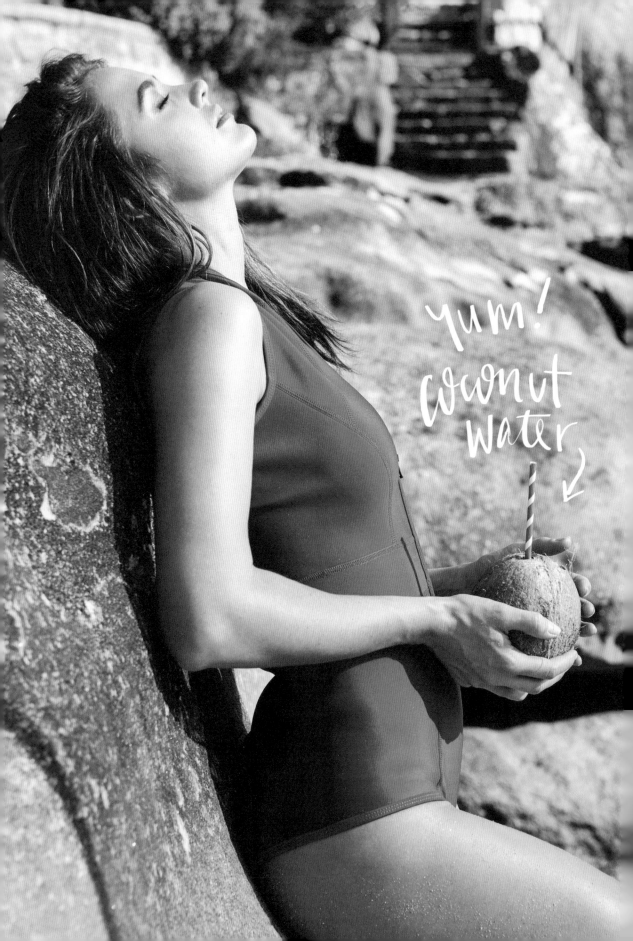

yum! coconut water

4. Rest is just as important as a workout

For many years I over-trained and didn't give my body much rest. This led to me feeling like I was constantly burning the candle at both ends. I would workout twice a day – it didn't matter how early or how late I finished work, I would go to the gym both before and after and feel so guilty if I didn't! I would rarely treat myself to massages or regular activities that relaxed both my mind and body, like yoga or a nice easy walk out in the fresh air.

My body is in the best shape it has ever been and it is because I have found a routine that works for me – and requires LESS working out (can you believe it?). That doesn't mean I don't work my butt off at the gym, it just means I train smarter and have incorporated balance into my weekly schedule.

Sharing my life with a professional athlete has taught me the importance of rest and recovery. For an athlete, their body is their most important career asset. If your body is not at its optimum, you will not be able to perform to your best potential and it can be the difference between winning or losing – it's that simple. Athletes take great care in not only how they train but also in how they recover. They listen to their bodies and do what they need to do to get themselves right, so that they can perform on the field week in and week out. Everyone should treat their bodies the way athletes do.

I have learnt to incorporate rest and recovery into my training schedule by structuring my workouts in a very simple way. I workout hard on one day, have an active recovery every alternate day and a FULL day of rest once or twice a week, depending on how I am feeling.

A workout day for me consists of a hard (usually cardio) one-hour session. This is either running or boxing based. An active recovery day is pilates or weights, both of which tone my body. On a workout day I leave the gym a hot sweaty mess, I push myself as hard as I can and make sure I leave nothing in the tank at the end. On my active recovery days, my heart rate is raised but I don't really sweat or get out of breath. On my rest days, I do ABSOLUTELY nothing. I enjoy movies or TV on the couch or a nice day out with friends or family. On these days I give my mind and body a complete rest, with no guilt. (You can see my 4-week training program on page 76.)

I have now learnt to LOVE my rest days and value how much healthier they have made me!

5. Mind & soul – keep tabs on your mental health

A big part of being healthy is awareness of your mental health. Make it a priority to ensure your emotional and mental health is in check. We are always encouraged to exercise, eat healthy and drink lots of water, but not many people talk about taking care of what goes on in our heads.

Due to my personal and highly publicised experiences with mental health and the fact that it is something that runs in my family, I don't have any fear of talking about it and being open about my mental health or helping those around me feel more comfortable talking about it.

Because there is such a stigma surrounding mental health, not many people even know where to begin when they're going through challenging times or how to help someone they know who is in a dark place.

Seeking professional help is paramount. The biggest misconceptions we have when we're struggling with mental health issues are that we can deal with it ourselves and that it will just go away. Neither of these are true, and in my experience the sooner you can talk to a professional about what you're going through, the better you will feel. There is nothing to be embarrassed or ashamed of – one in five Australians experience mental illness. It does not make you any less of a person; it does not make you incompetent or less worthy of any of life's joys. You are also not alone in your struggle, nor will you be on the journey by yourself. You will be surprised by how much support and care you will receive when you are open and honest with people. And if they're not understanding, then that is their loss in life, not yours!

Life shrinks or Expands in proportion to one's COURAGE.

-ANAÏS NIN

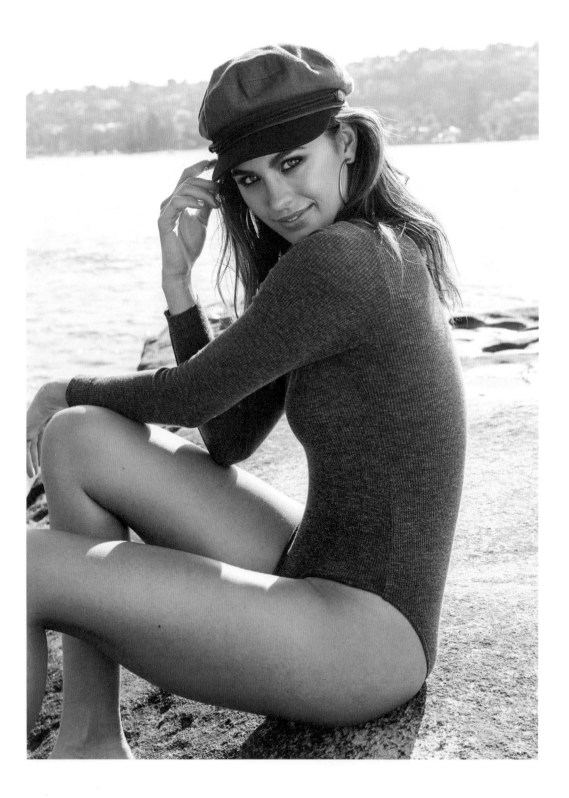

I am not ashamed to say that I see a professional regularly myself. I've found it really helpful and I feel so much better after a session. I get to download all my worries and stresses, and talk through ways in which I can communicate better, deal with stress, relax my mind and body more, and just feel mentally 'lighter'.

If you or someone you know is suffering, make sure you surround yourself with as much support as possible and work on a mental health plan or strategy to help you get back on track.

Please call LIFELINE 13 11 14 if you need help.

6. Keep it natural – being your own, unique 'cool'

I decided in my early teens that illicit drug use and binge drinking did not sit well with me. The idea of using drugs or alcohol as a stimulus to give me a high so I could have fun seemed disempowering. Although at the time I had tried neither, I felt deeply they had nothing of great value to add to my life or the lives of others. I learnt very quickly that this choice was a little out of the ordinary and would stand me apart from the 'cool' party crowd. Many in my industry believe having a good time goes hand in hand with taking drugs and getting drunk.

Today, ten years after making that decision, I am very proud to say I don't do drugs and never have. I have had many a fun night, though, and definitely enjoy a social drink or a wine with my meal and, yes, I have on the rare occasion had a few too many drinks. It comes down to your intention and this is where I see a difference between alcohol and drugs. When someone chooses to use a drug for recreational purposes, they do it to give themselves a high – the intent is clear! However, you can drink alcohol without getting drunk and without it changing your mood.

Now I do love to have fun, so part of the adventure of being different from the crowd has helped me define fun in ways I believe are more empowering and lead to a healthier body and mind. Finding my natural highs and keeping my unique 'cool' has helped me to grow as a person. Mostly I love to get outdoors in fresh air and be active. The sunshine has loads of feel-good energy-enhancing vitamin D in it, and keeping my body active keeps my mind fresh. Going for walks, swimming and doing outdoor activities are high on my list. But I encourage everyone to create their own healthy ways to have fun.

What has happened to me along the way is actually what has set me apart, and the things that often made me feel on the outside are now the very things that are serving me the most in life. The respect and admiration I have been shown for being true to myself has far outweighed the challenges. Our young people need more role models spreading a healthier message on fun, partying, drugs and drink, and I am passionate about spreading that message!

Everyone has their own pathway to follow and explore. Find your natural high . . . be uniquely cool!

7. Balance

Finding balance in your life is easier said than done. As soon as I left high school, I was so driven and determined to achieve my goals and dreams that I would work weekends and say yes to almost every career opportunity that came my way. My hours were often so long that I would always say no to going out and having fun with my mates. I missed a lot of my close friends' 21st birthdays and engagement parties, and one year I missed Easter with my family because I was working in Alice Springs. I was constantly on planes, in different states every other week. I worked out like crazy and rarely relaxed.

I don't ever regret how hard I worked as it has led me to where I am in life. A good work ethic is admirable. I still work hard, I don't think I will ever be able to not work, it is ingrained in me. The only thing that changed is that I am not as hard on myself. I have learnt that placing that amount of pressure on yourself is unhealthy.

Quality time with family and friends is invaluable and you should always make time for those who love and care for you. Don't be afraid to work your arse off, but don't forget to have fun and let your hair down. Success means nothing if you don't have people to share it with.

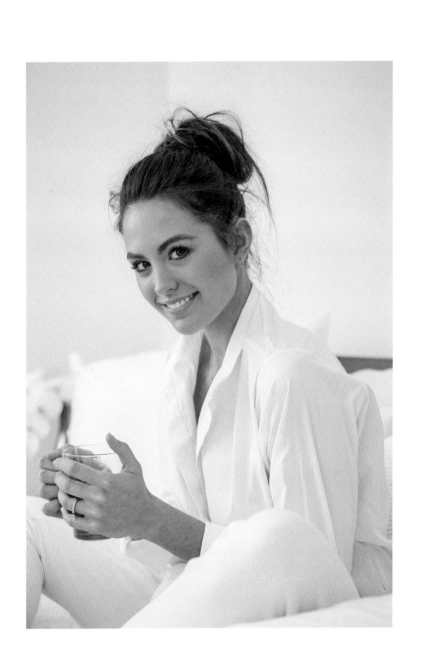

Sleep

Sleep is the most undervalued asset in life!

In this day and age, if someone asks you how you've been and you don't reply with 'Yeah, I've been soooo busy,' you're made to feel like you are underachieving. We push ourselves so much to be successful and achieve in all parts of our lives that we often forget to rest and give our bodies the chance to recharge.

I went through a stage in my career when I lived off three hours sleep per night and my health suffered significantly. My skin was terrible, I craved sugar all the time because I was low on energy, I kept getting sick and felt like I constantly had a cold.

There are still weeks in my life where I live off hardly any sleep. I have managed to balance this out, though, by ensuring this isn't a constant occurrence. I reduce the amount of exercise I do in these periods and drink lots of water. I also believe that power naps are incredible – I've done it on my lunch breaks and it has made the world of difference!

Everyone should aim for eight hours of sleep at night to maintain optimum health and wellness; no one likes a tired, grumpy person!

8. Be kind to yourself and others

A healthy body can be a size 6 or a size 16. Embrace what you have and learn to love your perfections and imperfections equally. You are unique; there is no one else like you in the whole wide world so why try to be someone you are not!

I believe in being the best version of yourself and living up to your potential. I believe in having role models and looking up to people who inspire you. But don't compare yourself to others – I find that whenever I do this, I forget about all the things I have achieved or the things that I love about myself. The most beautiful people are those who are happy and confident within themselves, not those who try to imitate others.

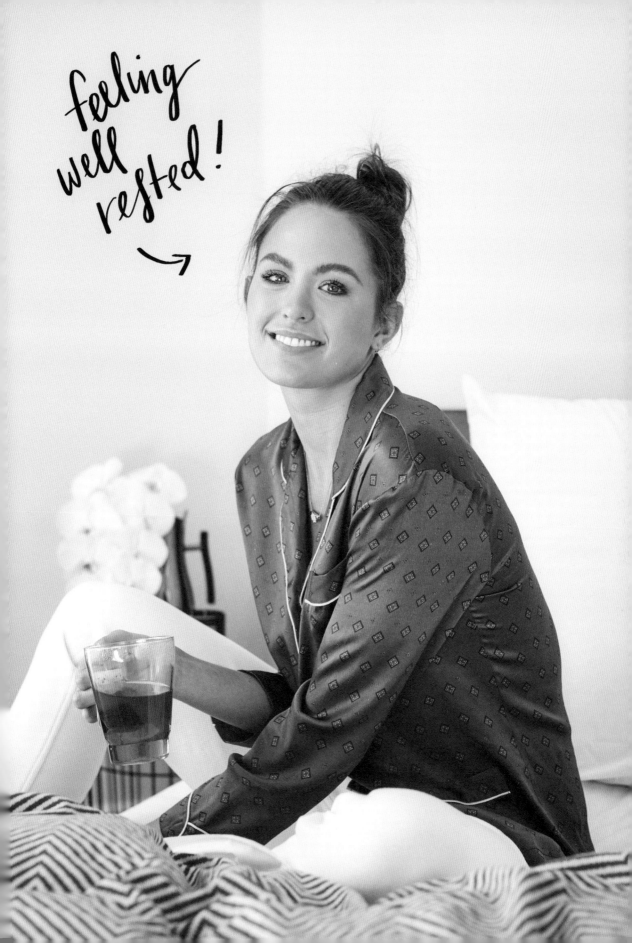

feeling
well
rested!

Supplements

I'M ALWAYS ASKED ABOUT supplements, what protein powders I use, what superfoods I add to my smoothies or what vitamins I'm taking.

The truth is, I've never really been into powders or supplements as I believe food can have all of the nutrients we require if we eat the right things in the right amounts.

I take fish oil, magnesium and turmeric most days because they work really well for my body. I only use superfood powders like spirulina or wheatgrass when I'm really struggling to fit enough greens into my diet. I believe that two big handfuls of baby spinach in my smoothie in the morning is better than a few scoops of a powdered substance. Protein powder has its place, but I've never really used it – I prefer to get my protein through my meals in the form of beans, legumes, eggs or meat.

However, in our busy lives it isn't always possible to prepare every single meal with all the protein and nutrient-dense fruit and vegetables we need to achieve optimum health. And this is where I have some little helpers stored away to assist me with making sure I'm eating as well as I can.

Spirulina

Dark in colour and sourced from the bottom of the ocean. Don't be put off by the not-so-great smell of this rich green powder; it is high in vegetable protein, vitamin B12 and minerals such as iron.

– –

Udo's oil

A mix of essential oils, including flaxseed oil, sesame oil, sunflower oil and coconut oil, Udo's oil is an excellent source of Omega 3 and antioxidants. Combine with some lemon juice, cracked pepper and sea salt and you have the ultimate salad dressing!

– –

Fish oil

My hair, skin and nails benefit so much from adding extra omegas to my nutrition plan. I always take fish oil in tablet form.

– –

Magnesium

When I'm exercising a lot or suffering from stress, I always up my intake of magnesium. I prefer to take it in powdered form; a teaspoon in water before bed helps to relax my muscles, reduce my stress and get me ready for sleep.

– –

Turmeric

Turmeric has so many potent anti-inflammatory qualities and is full of antioxidants! I include fresh or powdered turmeric in my veggie juices, add it to a tea or use it to spice up my meals. When I'm travelling and it's harder for me to include it in my diet, I take turmeric in tablet form.

What is turmeric? To put it simply, it is the spice that makes curries vibrantly yellow and it's used in a lot of Indian dishes. But I use it for medicinal purposes for my brain and body. For centuries turmeric has been used in Ayurvedic and Chinese medicines to treat a multitude of ailments. Besides being incredibly beneficial internally, turmeric's high level of antioxidants helps to fight free radicals, which assists in keeping your skin's elasticity and makes it glow from the inside out.

– –

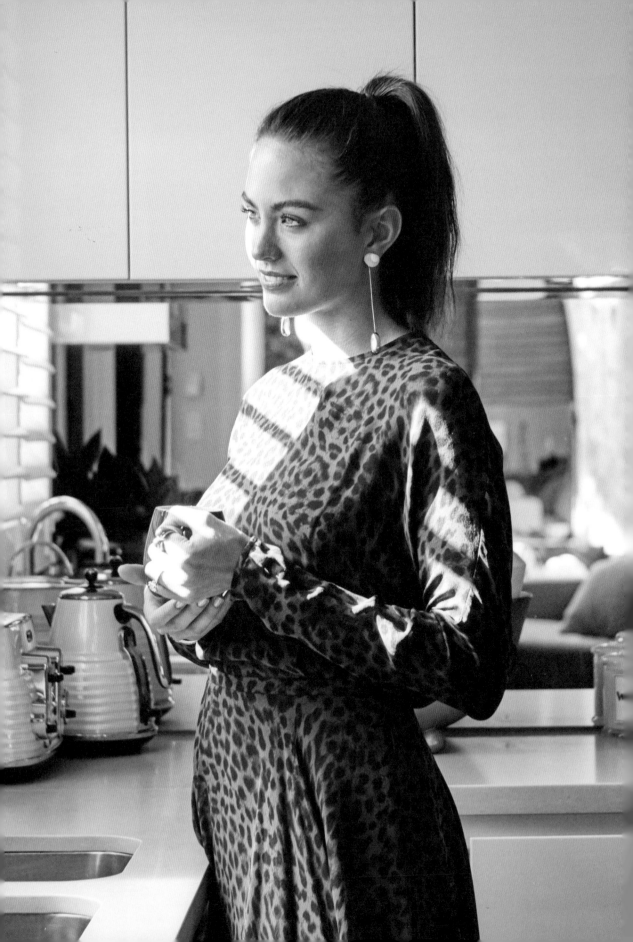

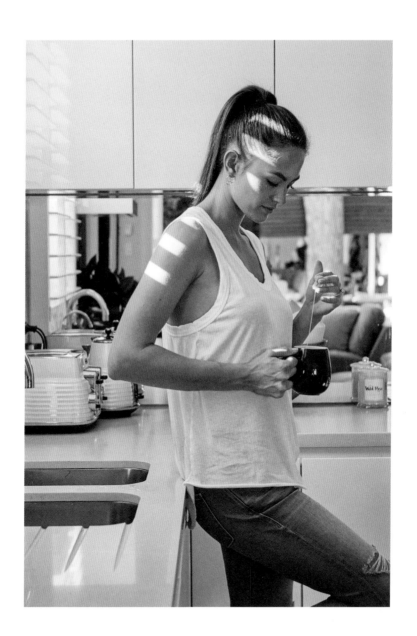

My morning routine

HAVING A MORNING ROUTINE is so important. For me, it ensures that I set the tone for the day and can get the most out of everything that I do.

I've always been an early riser. I find it difficult to sleep in and hate feeling like I have wasted a morning. I am at my most productive when I first wake up, I feel fresh and my head is full of thoughts and ideas.

As soon as I wake up, I make myself my morning elixir, Healing Turmeric Juice (see page 98). I feel like it cleanses and detoxes my digestive system and kickstarts my metabolism. I give myself fifteen minutes to sip on it and use that time to answer emails, check my schedule for the day – as sometimes call sheets or briefs can get updated late at night – and if I have the day off I write a to-do list so that I can be as productive as possible with my time.

If my call time isn't before 6.30am (sometimes it can be really early, the earliest from memory was 2.45am!), I will fit in some form of exercise. How much sleep I've had or how full-on my schedule is determines what kind of exercise I do. If I'm feeling fresh, I will box for an hour, go for a run or attend a cardio-based class. If I'm feeling low on energy, I will sometimes just stretch for half an hour or go for a walk in the fresh air to clear my head and ease into the day.

There is a significant difference in how I feel if I workout before going to work versus not doing anything. I often get asked what motivates me to get up so early or just to exercise in general. It's the feeling I get after I have sweated or moved my body – I feel like everything is working, I'm warmed up, my brain has started to wake up, I feel fresh and alert, I feel strong and it shakes off any sluggishness. All of those things inspire and motivate me when my alarm goes off and I'm cosy and comfy in bed. I want those good feelings.

Once I've completed my workout or activity for the morning, I have breakfast and go to work. Sometimes I eat brekky on the way to work or I eat when I'm getting my hair done on set. I rarely skip breakfast. If I do, I cannot keep up with my schedule. My job requires a lot of energy and for me to be switched on and focused at all times. I represent big companies and I always want to do the best job that I possibly can. I strive to execute all facets of my job at a professional and admirable level; I don't believe in shortcuts or getting something for nothing. I always want to be on my game!

Whatever your lifestyle or career, make sure you have a morning routine so that you give yourself the best opportunity to get the most out of your day. It can be simple and be just one thing you do for yourself before attending to your family or significant other. Tailor it to suit your needs and desires, and watch the difference it makes to your life when you begin your day with intent and purpose.

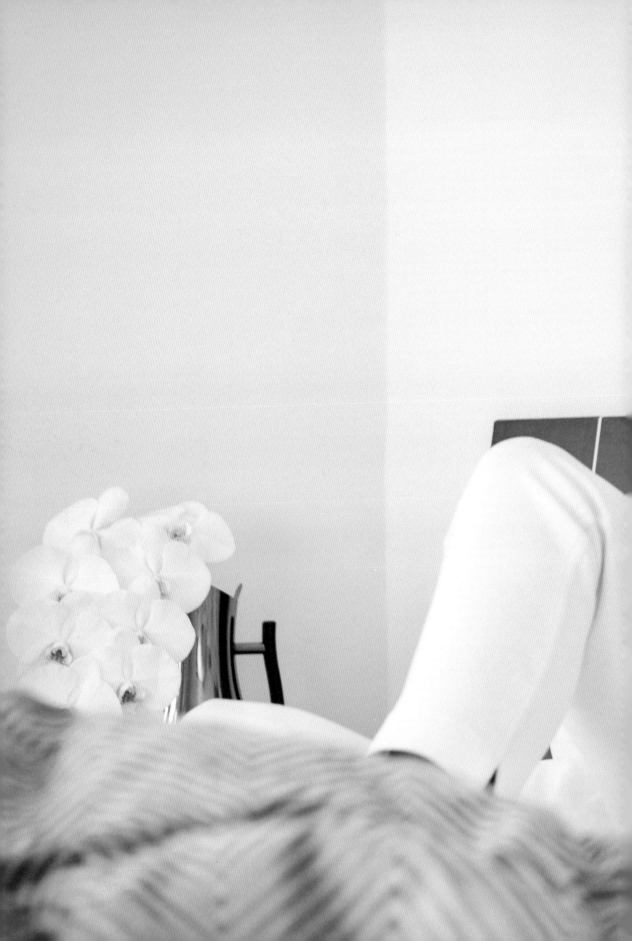

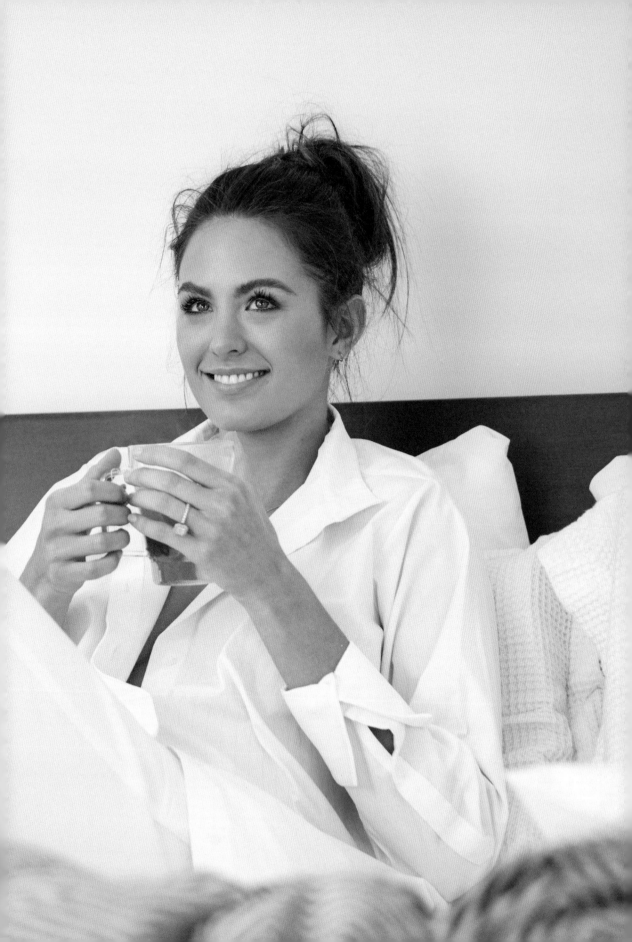

Peer pressure — stay true to who you are, always

I OFTEN GET ASKED what my greatest achievement is. At 25 I do feel as though I have done a lot in a short amount of time. Careerwise I have achieved many of the things I set out to do with MANY more things to accomplish. Personally I have grown and learnt so much since I graduated from high school as a bright-eyed young girl with big dreams and not a care in the world. I own property, I've built up a solid business, I'm engaged, and I absolutely love my work. But as I look at my personal and professional accomplishments, my greatest achievement is more of an internal one. I work in an industry that is incredibly cutthroat, full of rejection and external pressure. I've been in uncomfortable situations more times than I can count on two hands.

I've always felt a bit different. As a teenager I was the girl with the longest school skirt, I wore glasses and had braces, was teased for being studious and called a teacher's pet on numerous occasions. Unlike the popular girls, I didn't colour my hair or own any cool branded clothes or designer stuff. I didn't drink or smoke or experiment with drugs. I was never invited to any of the parties with the cool kids. My memory is crystal clear of one particular lunchtime at high school; a group of us were sitting around in a circle near the assembly area. We all used to sit in big circles and eat at recess or lunch, as the tables were always dibbed first by the senior students. One of our year's 'popular' pretty girls approached our small lunch group, her two sidekicks in tow. She started talking about how her birthday was coming up and she was going to have an awesome party at her house. Then she began to hand out the pink printed invites that were folded once over. She went around to everyone in the group, making quite a show out of it, and when it came to me, the last girl in the circle, she turned her back, faced the rest of the girls and said, 'See you all there, it's going to be so much fun,' and walked off, leaving me invite-less and embarrassed. I remember feeling so small that day. I cried when I got home from school. I knew I hadn't been invited because I didn't drink and wasn't cool and would have been seen as a downer at the party. I was only fifteen.

It was at high school that I learnt one of the greatest lessons life has ever taught me: never to succumb to any of the external pressures that are placed on me.

And despite how glamorous my life now appears to be from the outside, just like at high school, I still refuse to change who I am and what I believe in to fit with a certain group or do things that are considered cool.

That is my greatest achievement – not once have I altered my core values or beliefs to fit into my industry or social setting. And I am proud of that.

Too often I see young women try to morph themselves into something they are not for nothing more than acceptance. To please a guy, to look good in a dress they saw in a magazine, to look like the bikini girl on Instagram, to get invited to 'that' event. If there is one thing I can assure you of, it's that the people who truly love and care for you in life will admire you more for being genuine, authentic and true to your own self-worth rather than changing who you are to fit into society's or an individual's ideals.

The things that set me apart as a teenager, the things that often left me feeling alone and rejected, are now the things that serve me best in life.

The pageant that changed my universe

MISS UNIVERSE CHANGED MY life. If I didn't take the chance and enter the pageant, I can safely say that my career wouldn't be where it is today. It is an opportunity I am so grateful for and to this day the memories from my time spent competing in the beauty pageant still bring a smile to my face.

I actually wasn't going to write about my time in Miss Universe in this book. I eventually decided to write about the pageant because it was such a big moment in my life and what goes on behind the sparkles, spray tans and bikinis is rarely spoken about.

So let's start at the beginning . . . In 2010 I was living in Sydney. I was coming in to my second year living away from home, still finding my feet, getting my groove and becoming used to having an independent life. I had spent 2009 studying acting in Sydney, modelling in Shanghai and working in a bar four nights a week to help pay the rent. Back in those days I was living week to week. I had moved from the Gold Coast to Sydney on a one-way plane ticket, with $700 in my bank account and all my belongings packed into a suitcase. Some weeks after I had paid my rent, my acting tuition and any other bills I had, I would have so little to spend on groceries that a packet of apples and a few tins of tuna would have to get me by until my next paycheck.

After a year of living like this, I had started to dream up a little plan. I had taken the chance of moving to Sydney with the goal of breaking into the entertainment industry. I'd always loved the thrill of performing or being in front of a camera, and I possessed

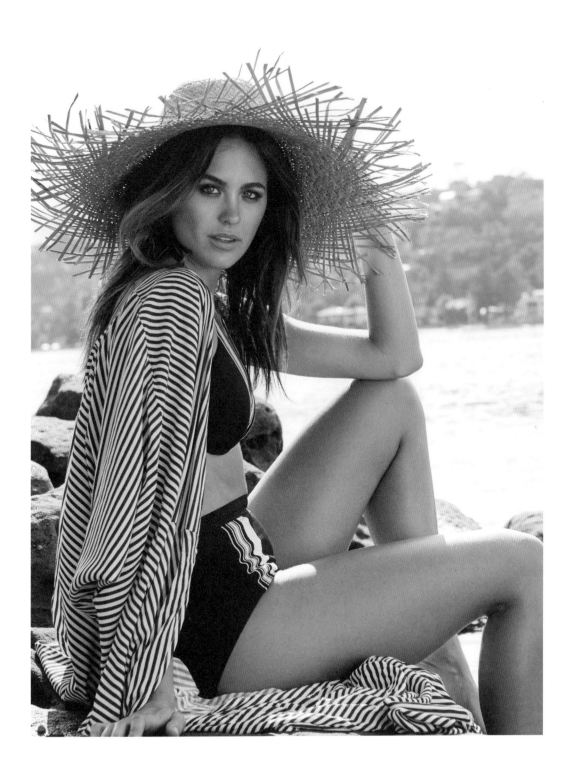

a genuine desire to use my career to give back to the community and engage myself in lots of charity work. Between working and studying, I would volunteer some of my free time at the city's homeless shelters; I found that extremely rewarding and it only fuelled my desire to help others even more.

When the opportunity to enter Miss Universe came across my path, I eagerly filled out the registration papers and applied. I had closely watched Rachael Finch's pageant journey. We were both Queensland girls and had crossed paths numerous times at various fashion events. The modelling industry is quite small so you often get to know all the other girls well; you're standing in lines for hours at castings or booked for the same shows together. So seeing fellow model Rachael enter and win the beauty contest definitely inspired me to enter.

Before this, beauty pageants hadn't been my thing; I hadn't grown up with a dream to be Miss Universe, nor had I really prepared myself before I entered. Besides working part-time as a model for the previous twelve months, I had had no real experience of doing my own hair or makeup, and walking in high heels was still uncomfortable for me. I had no idea what pageants truly involved, and I did not like sparkles or glitz or any sort of glamour and would never have dreamt of putting a hair extension anywhere near my head. It was safe to say that if I was a filly entering the Melbourne Cup, all the odds were against me so when I rocked up to the pageant registration day, no one would have backed me to win the race – not even me.

Initially, my idea was to enter Miss Universe Australia, see how far into the audition process I could go, have some fun, meet new people and, most importantly, suss out how the competition worked so I could come back in a couple of years' time and give it a really good crack. I was only eighteen years old so I had no intention or expectation of progressing too far in the competition. I really just wanted to use the opportunity to practise talking on a stage in front of a crowd, really hone in on my public speaking skills, become confident walking in a ball gown and a bikini, and I was curious to see how the crazy world of beauty pageants works . . . I soon learnt it only becomes crazier as it goes on but I'll get to that later!

Each state around Australia holds a registration day and then the girls who get through are divided up into groups who compete in heats in their home state. Even though I was a Queensland girl, I was living in Sydney at the time so I represented New South Wales. The heats were all held at shopping centres so I very quickly got used to being in front of a crowd of strangers. But the first few times I was in my bikini I nearly died from the nerves, I was so far out of my comfort zone it was scary.

I ended up harnessing those nerves, though, and after five rounds of heats over just as many months, I somehow progressed to the final of Miss Universe Australia.

I don't say somehow lightly, either. Some of the girls who had entered were extremely serious about it, they had been training for months with pageant trainers (yes, they do exist!), rehearsing answers to the infamous pageant questions, practising their catwalk routines, studying poses, and spending fortunes on gowns, bikinis, makeup and hair. I was an eighteen-year-old with absolutely no idea about any of it and wore the same pair of heels for the entire process of the heats because that's all I had and all I could afford. In hindsight, it was hilarious that I even entered so underprepared.

Three nights before the final and I get a phone call from the assistant to the pageant director. She spends half an hour talking to me about where I'm from, what I've done, whether or not I had a boyfriend or a serious relationship, what my family is like, where I went to school. It was after this conversation that I knew I should probably get a really nice dress for the finals so I called Mum straight away. None of my family were even planning to be at the event as I had told them that I probably wasn't going to place, but I was having an amazing time and loving the experience so I wasn't fussed.

Mum ended up flying down as I had two full days of rehearsals and needed someone to help me get the dress and buy some jewellery. I recall so vividly Mum coming to bring me lunch in one of the rehearsal breaks the day before the final. All of the girls were around and I introduced some of them to my mum. When I got home that night, Mum said to me, 'Jesinta, I just want you to know that all of those girls are really beautiful. Like, really, really

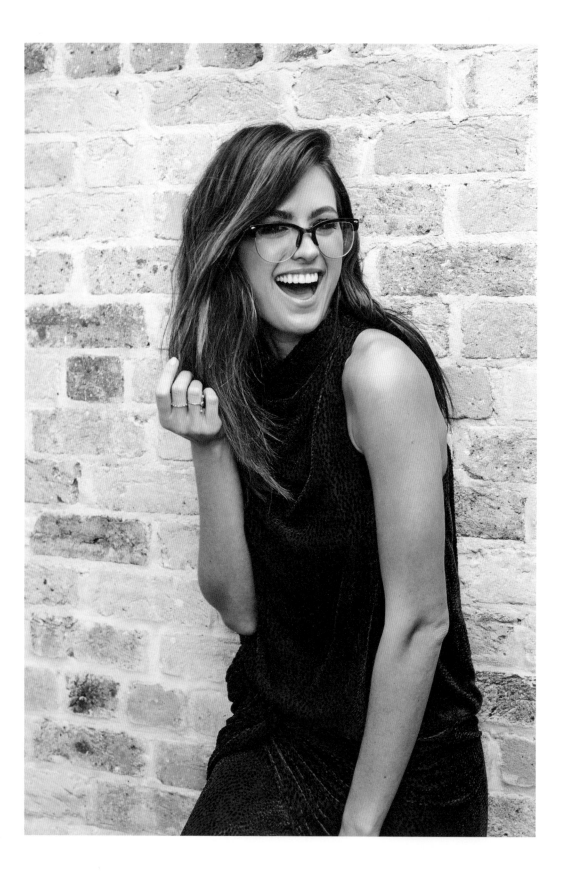

beautiful. I don't want you to get your hopes up too much, I mean they are just stunning.'

Nothing like a good little chat from your own mother to bring you back to earth. I love her attitude and approach to life, she doesn't sugarcoat anything and to this day we always laugh about this little moment we had together.

The night of the Miss Universe Australia final had come so quickly, the show is so nerve-racking that it all happened in a bit of whirl. After progressing through the rounds and stumbling on my final question, the next thing I remember there was gold confetti flying all around me, some got stuck in my eye – it's the only thing I can attribute to me crying like a true beauty queen cliché. 😄 They had placed the crown on my head and a bouquet of red roses in my arms. Some crazy lady on a phone was also screaming 'She won! She won!' as she ran around the room. One can only assume that was my mum, who didn't think I was beautiful enough to win the competition; shock does funny things to people.

I was immediately whisked off stage by a security guard and led down a walkway where it was so dark I was finding it hard not to trip over my own feet, then told to wait beside a door. The pageant director hurried over and told me that I was about to walk into a media conference. 'Just say you can't wait to represent Australia overseas and this is an honour,' she said as she opened the door and pushed me through.

Flashing lights instantly blinded me, someone grabbed me by the arm and placed me on a stool in front of a Miss Universe banner. Questions were being fired at me from every direction; I had hardly answered one before being asked another. The weirdest question I got asked that night from someone who I can only assume was an independent freelance journalist was, 'Do you believe in God?' That was my introduction to the craziness of the media and what life was going to be like living in the spotlight.

I drove home that night, in my ball gown in my little Toyota Yaris, which I was slowly paying off week by week. Mum and I ate leftovers for dinner in my cramped studio apartment where I could almost stir a pot on the stove while I was having a shower. There was only one bed so Mum and I crashed together, absolutely exhausted. We had a 5am start the next day for all my interviews with Australia's favourite morning shows.

The next six weeks went so quickly and before I knew it I was jetting off to Las Vegas to represent Australia in the international Miss Universe pageant.

Most people don't realise that all the girls arrive three weeks before the big night and you spend every single day rehearsing, filming, attending events and working for charity. This gives the organisation time to interview all of the 80-plus contestants and get to know them thoroughly before determining the winner, who will travel the world and represent the pageant for the next twelve months. Basically, it's like a three-week long job interview!

Behind the scenes – what Miss Universe is really like

The competition is ON as soon as you step off the plane. I thought the girls in the Australian competition took it seriously, but this was another level. I have honestly never seen women so perfectly put together in my life. Not a single strand of hair was out of place, the tans, makeup and nails were immaculate. I soon learnt that some countries take so much pride in a competition like Miss Universe that their entrants have spent half their lives in preparation for it. From early on, these girls enter into training and some even go into 'pageant houses' where they are taught everything about pageant life. Before they fly out to the pageant, they have every single outfit for every day planned, along with how they will do their hair and makeup each day – their preparation is a full-time job and for some women it is the opportunity to start a new life. With more than 80 countries involved, not everyone has had a privileged upbringing or lives in a stable country or city, so for some it is the chance to break away.

The first day is the most daunting. You are divided into groups of four and each group has their own chaperone. The chaperones are older ladies who become like a mum for you. After some time, many girls become homesick and there are usually tears and often a big, squishy hug from your chaperone makes it all better.

I was placed in a group with Miss Brazil, Miss Great Britain and Miss Guam, who was also my roomie. Our chaperones or anyone from the organisation were not allowed to call us by our first names, as it could show favouritism, so we were just known by our countries. Even to this day whenever I chat to any of the girls, they still refer to me as 'Aussie'.

I was so lucky to have such a friendly, fun and chilled-out roommate. Guam had the same approach as me – we were there to represent our countries the best we could and have fun along the way. We weren't fiercely competitive, so we weren't going to be putting itching powder in each other's clothes or marbles on the bathroom floor (by the way, that kind of cattiness only exists in the movies).

I ended up bonding with so many of the girls during the three weeks. Miss Ireland and I became really close, she was the favourite to take the crown on the final night. We shared the same sense of humour, we would spend our days laughing and giggling at silly jokes. Whenever we had to pair up with another contestant in an activity or group event, Miss Ireland and I made sure we were together. We still keep in touch.

The pageant is a crazy little world; as soon as the girls arrive to compete, there are huge international blogs that start trying to pick the top 15, 10, 5 and the winner. Every photo from your professional photo shoot and rehearsals, and anything uploaded to social media (which was only Twitter and Facebook because Instagram wasn't popular in 2010), was grabbed by these blogs and people would start to vote online and begin to determine favourites. None of this had anything to do with the pageant, nor did it influence the results; however, it was talked about a lot among all of us and we knew exactly where each of us sat with the Miss Universe fans.

Before I got to Vegas, I had no idea about the scale of the competition. It is the second most viewed event on international television behind the football World Cup. There were fans who had flown in from around the world and booked hotel rooms in Vegas, knowing that all the contestants would be there for weeks before the final show. They would be waiting in hotel foyers, some with signs with your name written on it and cut-outs of your face on t-shirts. For this reason we constantly had bodyguards with us, we could not leave our rooms without our chaperone or a bodyguard and always travelled in our groups – and you had to wear your sash at all times!

I had the time of my life over those three weeks. Each morning, all the 80-plus contestants had breakfast together in our hotel and I used that time to get to know everyone. The worst part about those mornings was the fact you were at a buffet and if you have ever been to Vegas you will know what I mean when I say the buffets are HUGE. All of us had been watching what we were eating in the weeks leading up to Vegas and all of a sudden we had every single food on earth available to us, en masse. Think waffles, pancakes, pikelets and every topping or condiment you can possibly imagine, plus more, true American style. Self-control of the highest order had to be exercised over the whole three weeks.

I remember one contestant really enjoying herself at the buffet breakfasts most mornings and, when her pageant director arrived a few days before the final, she got in trouble. We all felt really sorry for her; all the girls rallied around and supported her. Pageant directors can be really full-on, their job and reputation relies on how well their contestant does in the pageant so they want to make sure everything is in order for the best chance at winning. This includes watching what you eat and being in the best shape possible.

The camaraderie and friendship I had developed with the girls during my time in Vegas really shone through a few days before the show. Back home, my pageant director had commissioned a particular dress for me to wear if I made it through to the eveningwear section of the competition. Each section is scored out of ten by the panel of judges and the highest scoring girls progress to the next round. My evening dress didn't fit me well, it had been made poorly and I knew that if I did make it to the eveningwear section and I wore that dress, I would not make it through to the next round.

I expressed my concerns to Miss Ireland who had become like a sister to me. I tried on the dress for her and did a few walks up and down the hotel corridor and she agreed that I could not wear it on stage. She took me to her room and told me she had two dresses, as she hadn't decided which one to wear on the night and wanted a backup just in case. She offered one of her dresses to me to wear on the night. I had been so stressed and nervous up until this point and she instantly made me feel amazing. Her kindness blew me away and I will never forget that. She taught me a great lesson in the importance of the sisterhood and why we should always seek to help one another – acts of kindness stay with people forever and you should always take the opportunity to make someone's day a little bit brighter.

Comparing when I first arrived in Vegas and the night of the show, my thinking and attitude changed so much around beauty and what it meant to be beautiful. At first I was so overwhelmed by everyone's appearances and the illusion of perfection that I instantly put all of the women on pedestals. Look at her eyes, OMG her hair is amazing, her body is so toned and perfect, her legs are so long, her outfits are fantastic, etc., etc. What started to happen as the competition progressed was fascinating – my view about who I thought was physically more attractive started to change dramatically the more I got to know each person. The stories about their families or their jobs (some women were doctors, police officers or paramedics), what they stood for, what they believed in, what their dreams were for the future, all started to build up and create a depth around who they were as individuals. I was so intimidated by some of these girls when I first arrived, I felt nervous being around them and I questioned my place in the competition. Why was I there? How could I be so stupid to enter something which was so far out of my league?

However, who I thought was the most beautiful when I first arrived had changed completely by the time I left, and it taught me that true beauty lies beyond how someone physically appears – the most beautiful people I have encountered in my life are beautiful not because of how they look, but because of who they are.

opportunities do not wait.

-GREEK PROVERB

Listen to others but be your own person

THROUGH LIFE AND BUSINESS, the greatest things I have learnt are to ask questions and to listen.

I've always been inquisitive and loved to ask people about their stories, where they are from, what they do and how they have got to where they are today. I try to absorb as much information from people around me as possible. I've never pretended to know it all and I have always believed we should never stop learning. I've received some of the best advice and inspiration from asking questions and being interested in other people's lives or careers.

When you're a young woman, people will always want to tell you how things should be done – what you should be studying, who you should be dating, *how* you should be dating, how to do your job, how *not* to do your job. You can either be frustrated by this or use it as an opportunity to learn something and apply it to your life. Sometimes the best advice I've received has been the hardest to take, that's often when I know I should take more notice and listen closer to whatever I am being told. Feeling uncomfortable or confronted is often a good thing because it can spark change and transformation.

My advice to all young women is to always listen to what people around you have to say, but be your own person. No two lives are the same and you have to carve out a path for yourself using other people's wisdom, knowledge and advice as the tools to guide you – but not carry you – through life.

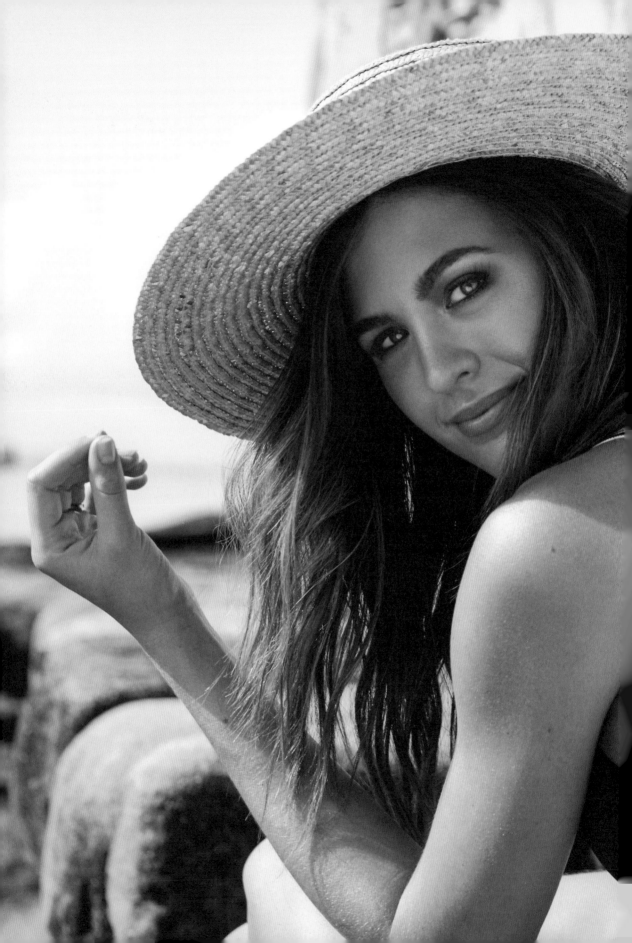

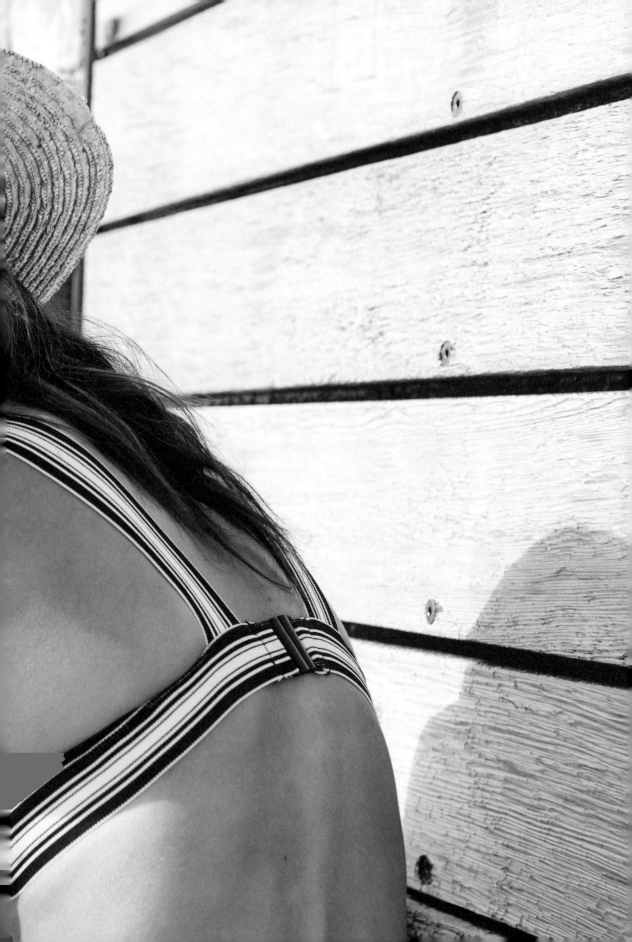

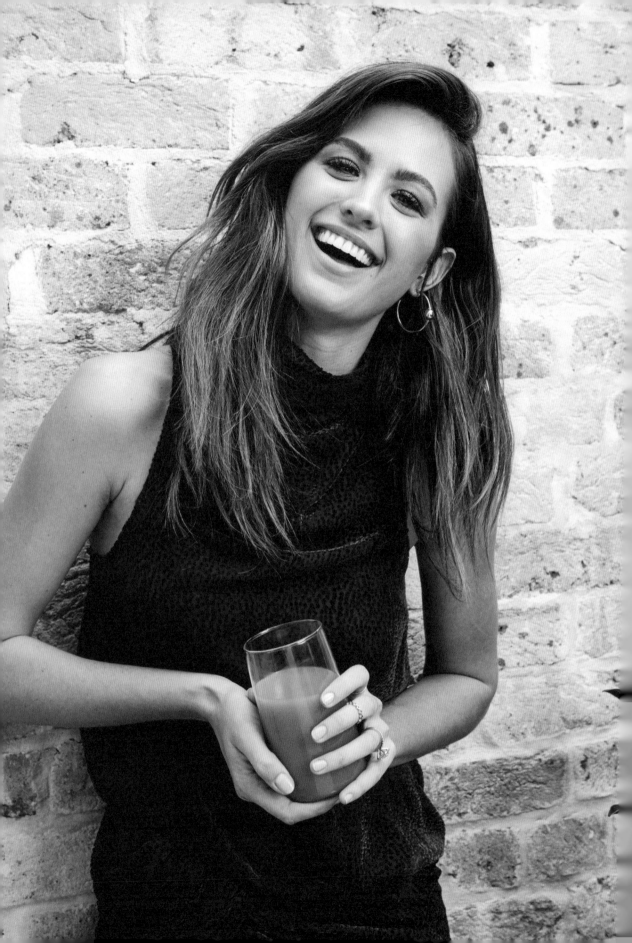

The sisterhood

WOMEN HAVE A VERY special bond with one another. Throughout history we have had to fight for our rights, protest for our equality and speak up when we didn't even have a voice.

Living in Australia in this century, I have to constantly remind myself of the heartbreaking hardships the women before me had to withstand and the struggle and fight they put forward to grant us the freedoms and independence we have today. I am always aware of where we have come from. Every time I vote, make a medical decision for myself, enrol in something educational or simply choose what it is that I want to wear for the day, I am grateful. Grateful because I can make my own choices which I may not have had the right to make 30 or 50 years ago as a woman. And while I have never felt like my gender has been a hindrance in my career or life, I can't help but think about other women on a global scale who still have to fight for their rights.

I believe in equality for all human beings; all races, all religions and all genders. Every human being needs to be treated with equal respect and dignity. Women and men should have the same pay if both are equally qualified and capable of doing a job. Women and men should both be able to vote with equal rights, and make the same medical and educational decisions without being hindered by gender.

I also believe that people in same-sex relationships should have the same rights to marriage and family as heterosexual couples.

My fight is one of equality across the board. No one should be made to feel less of a person or should have their quality of life diminished because of the colour of their skin, their origin, religion, sexual preference or gender.

Beauty

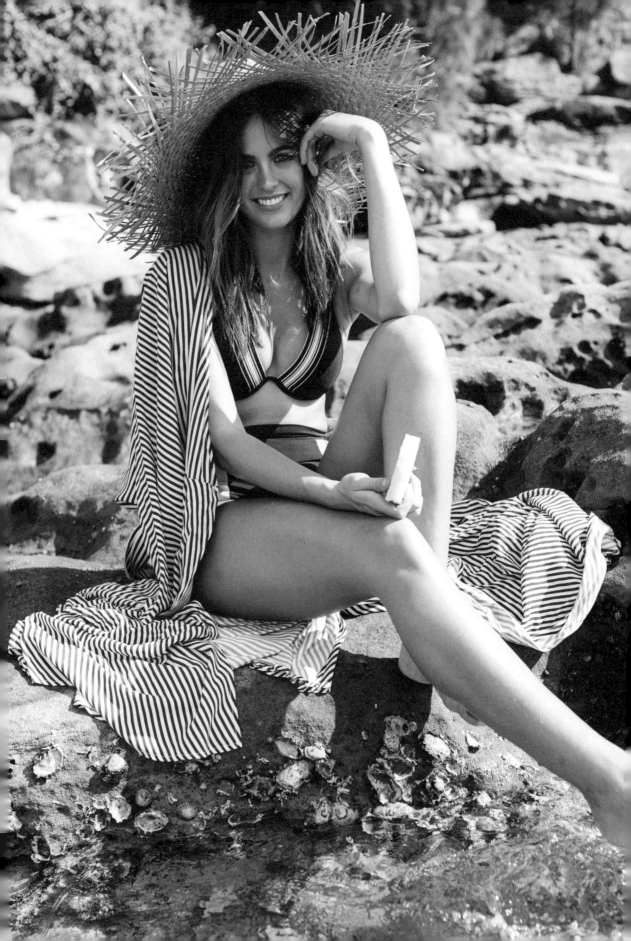

The importance of a consistent beauty routine

AS A TEENAGER I had great skin. I had the odd pimple that would raise its ugly head the night before an exam but other than that I didn't have too many skin troubles.

When I reached nineteen, everything changed. I developed really bad hormonal breakouts all around my jawline and on my cheeks. It was painful, red and no amount of makeup could hide it. My life had just begun to become public; I was frequently doing photo shoots and TV appearances. I remember being constantly embarrassed by my skin and some nights I would cry and cry because I didn't know how I was going to get up the next day and go to work feeling so incredibly insecure and self-conscious about the way I looked. I would try to conceal my breakouts before I would have to sit in the hair and makeup chair. My heart rate would instantly rise when the makeup artist would come at me with wipes as I was so nervous about someone seeing me bare faced. It had a significant impact on my self-esteem and I would have done absolutely anything to get rid of it.

I battled with bad skin for nearly two years, no product or facial seemed to work for me, and sometimes I felt like the more I tried to fix it, the worse it got.

Unfortunately for me it was a hormonal issue, and instead of going through that stage in my early teens, it hit me when I was in my late teens and early twenties. The embarrassment and shame I felt from having terrible skin has made me appreciate and also develop a consistent skincare routine that I stick to religiously. It doesn't matter if I'm on a plane or in another country; I always make it my priority to take care of my skin.

I am so lucky now, my skin is clear and I often get makeup artists commenting on how smooth and clean it is. Here are some tips to maintaining beautiful skin:

- Cleanse and moisturise every morning and nitght.

- Never sleep with your makeup on – EVER!

- Use a different moisturiser for morning and night. Night-time moisturiser should be richer so you wake up hydrated.

- Do not over-exfoliate. This can create more breakouts.

- Don't squeeze your pimples. Put some toothpaste on them before you go to bed to help dry them out.

- Invest in good quality products.

- Treat yourself to a facial occasionally.

- Be consistent.

If you're struggling with breakouts or acne, assess your diet, stress levels, how much you are sleeping and how much water you are drinking. Book an appointment with a healthcare professional and ask them to check your hormones. If they are unbalanced, work with someone to create more synergy within your body. When everything is more balanced in your life, there is less stress in your body so things like bad skin may calm down.

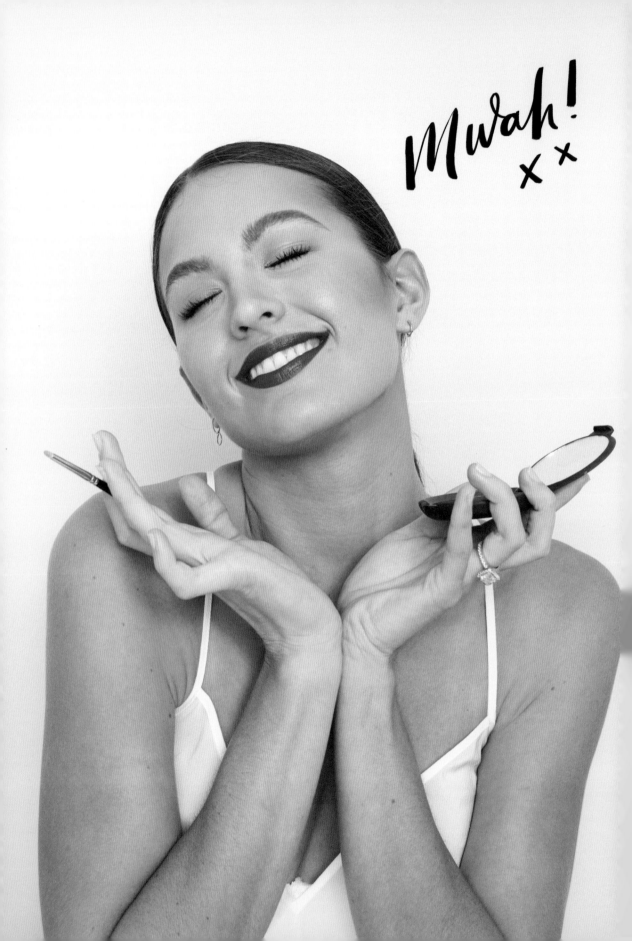

Mwah!
xx

My best makeup tips

MAKEUP IS A WONDERFUL way to express yourself and be playful – don't be afraid to try new things! I love experimenting with makeup and because of my job I'm always getting great tips and tricks from some of the best makeup artists in the country. If you're not sure where to begin, visit a cosmetics store or the beauty counter at a large department store to get you started.

Contour

Contouring has become the biggest beauty trend; it can define and refine your features. The contouring we see now in magazines is very heavy and requires lots of makeup to make it work. It's a technique that most makeup artists use on set for photo shoots and red carpet appearances rather than for everyday. I've adapted it into a more achievable daytime look that I love to use for business meetings or for a special outing.

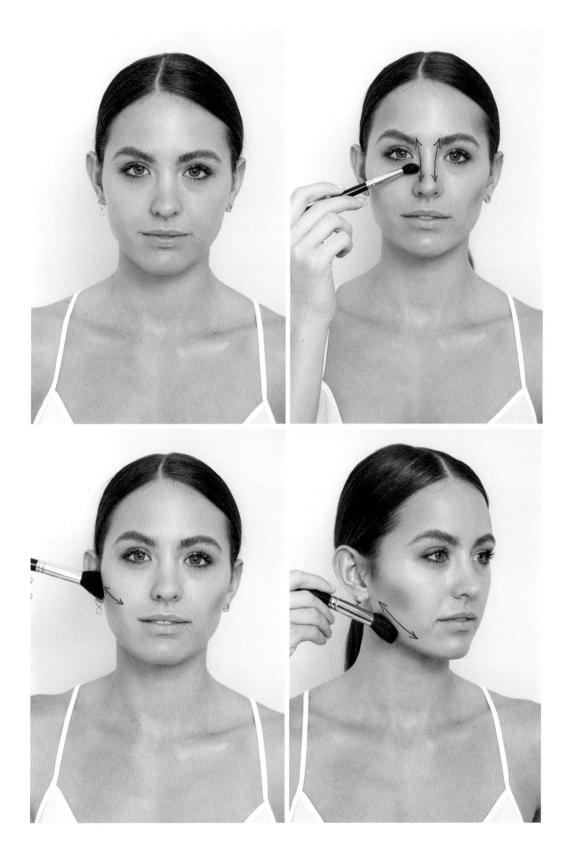

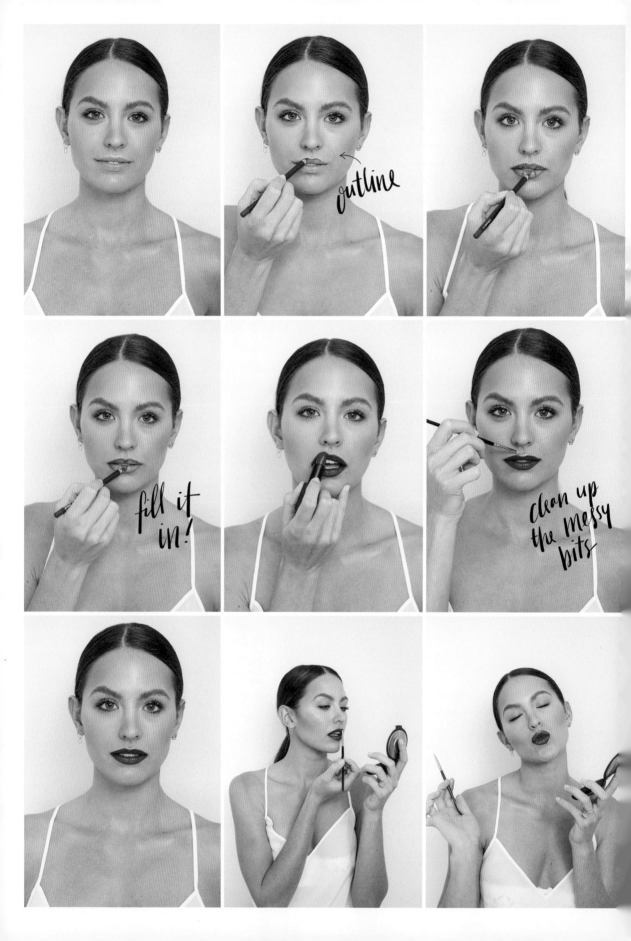

outline

fill it in!

clean up the messy bits

Red lip

A red lip makes me instantly feel glamorous. If you know how to do red lips properly, it will not only last all day or night, it is also the easiest way to take your makeup to the next level and make you look red-carpet ready. A lip liner, concealer, powder and the right shade of red for your skin tone is all you need to perfect this look.

Highlighter

I always highlight – if you know where to apply it, it can enhance the colour of your eyes, make your lips look plumper and enhance your cheekbones. Here is my beauty breakdown on highlighter.

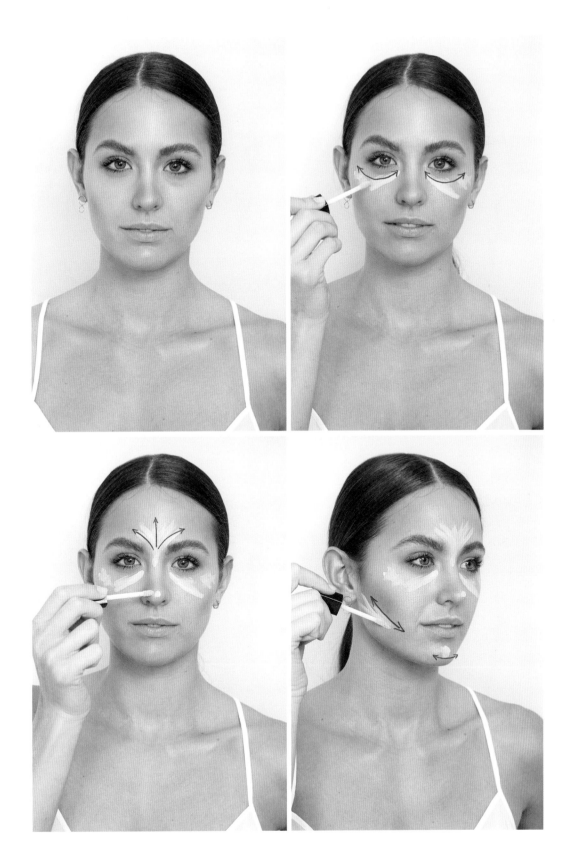

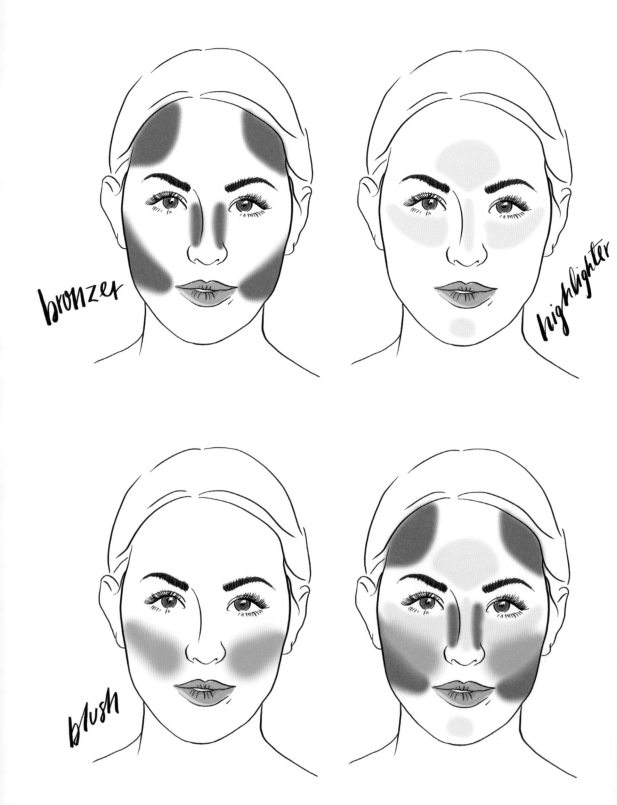

Where to apply your makeup

Knowing where to apply your blush, bronzer and other products can all get a bit confusing. Here's a simple diagram that will help.

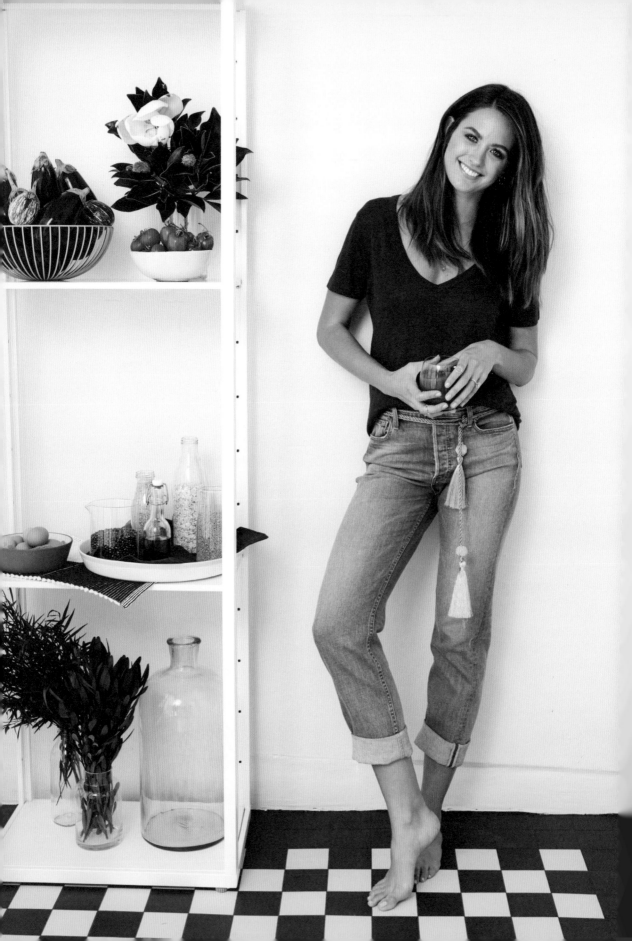

What causes bad skin

When my skin is not at its best, these things are usually to blame:

- Stress and anxiety.

- Gut health.

- Hormonal imbalance.

- Diet and lifestyle.

Reducing stress in your life is often hard and it has to be something that you are conscious about. Create a plan around doing things that physically and mentally relax you; you have to be proactive with it.

Acupuncture and exercise are two things that I find really helpful. Exercise always makes me feel better. Acupuncture has so many amazing health benefits; it works for some and not for others, though, so try it out and see if it's for you. An acupuncturist can specifically treat your health issues, and if you want them to focus on your skin, let them know. They will usually give you some supplements to also assist with this – these can be amazing!

Regular facials

While your skin is sensitive, minimise how much you touch it. Sometimes getting treatments too regularly can aggravate and increase the inflammation of your skin. Get the opinion of a few beauticians and come up with a plan that you stick to. Opt for something on the more gentle side; you don't want anything too full-on that will set you back.

Once a month I have a big clean, which is quite clinical and very specific to the needs of my skin. Then once a fortnight I have a facial that cleans my skin but is also a relaxing experience where I get a bit of a massage, the room is filled with candles and it completely relaxes my mind and body.

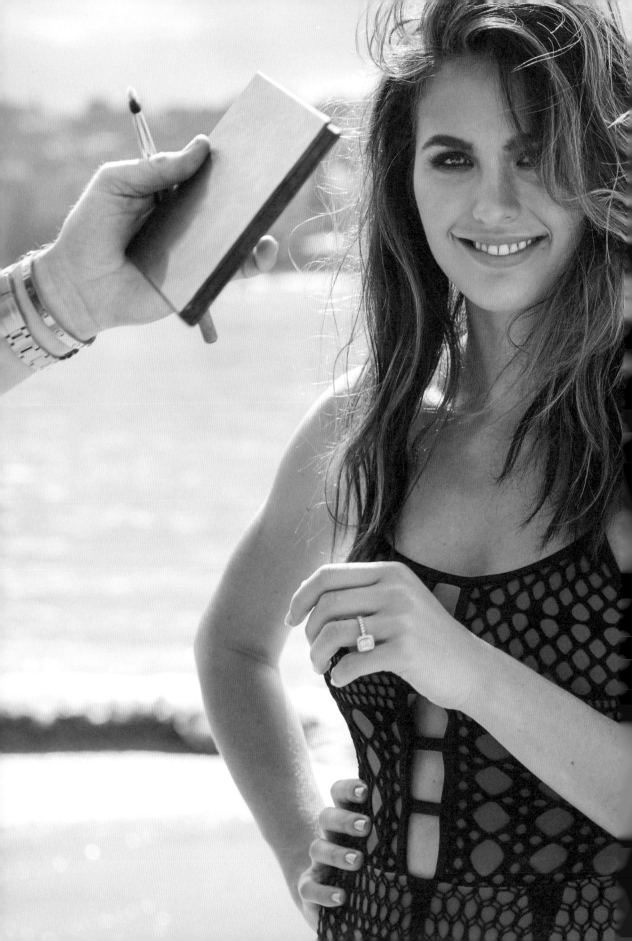

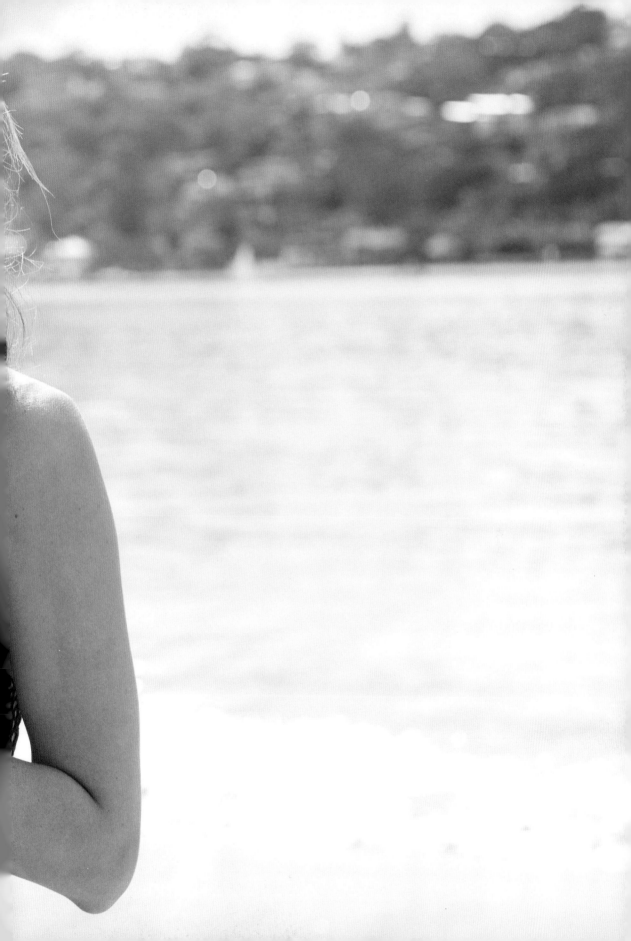

Diet and digestive health

I start every morning with warm water and lemon. Drink this before you eat anything. It detoxifies and kickstarts your digestive system.

Reduce sugar and alcohol in your diet; give your body a break and the chance to start healing. It's hard but start with something small, like no alcohol from Monday to Friday. Then if you can, do a two-week or, even better, three-week detox where you eliminate alcohol for that entire period of time.

Take turmeric and black pepper tablets every day. Turmeric works on reducing the inflammation in your body and the black pepper helps the body to absorb the turmeric properly.

Drink between 1.5 and 3 litres of water per day – this flushes the system and keeps your skin hydrated! Keep a bottle of water with you at all times; on your desk at work, in your handbag or your car. Draw little lines on the bottle with texta and write times on it then make sure you drink to that line at the right time. It will eventually create a habit.

Skin routine

Keep your skincare routine super simple. Don't use products that overstimulate or irritate the skin. The more basic products are usually the best. You don't need to spend a lot of money on fancy or high-end products.

Because I am so stringent with my skincare routine, I do have lots of products at home in my bathroom. I have the base products, which I absolutely love; however, I'm not afraid to try new things or change it up. I combine both natural and non-natural products. I sometimes even create my own stuff that I use on my face and body. I wear a mineral makeup instead of liquid when I'm not at work; I find my skin breathes so much better.

And remember, never sleep or workout with makeup on!

Gua sha — how to achieve healthy, glowing skin

My best friend Elliot shared the magic of *gua sha* with me after he learnt about it on a trip to Fiji. It is by far my favourite beauty secret and I am so excited to share it with you!

Gua sha is an ancient practice that has been used for centuries to cleanse the body. It was prominent in ancient Egyptian, Greek and Asian cultures and it has even been said the world's most beautiful woman, Cleopatra, used this method to clean her skin.

The first time I tried this method my skin was incredibly silky smooth for days afterwards; it was brighter and everyone would comment on my complexion. I have never used an exfoliant or product that compares to this amazing at-home treatment.

Your skin is your largest organ, and every day it comes into contact with so many different things, from perfumes and moisturisers, to pollution, toxins and all different sorts of fabrics. When you wash your body with soap and water, you only ever remove what is sitting on the surface of your skin; you can never permeate into the deeper layers of your skin so you are never truly cleansing it.

When you apply a *gua sha*, you are accessing right through the layers of skin to give you an amazing cleanse and a chance to get rid of toxins that may be deep within those layers.

If you are prone to breakouts, this will help you achieve amazing results. It aids in removing the bacteria in your skin, which reduces the amount of breakouts you get.

I wish I had been savvy to *gua sha* when I was in my late teens! I had terrible acne and I know this would have been really helpful to me. I hope by sharing this it helps someone who may be suffering from acne on their body or their face.

Although I prefer to only use *gua sha* on my body, you can also use it on your face — it really is a deep cleanse like no other that will leave your skin feeling extremely clean.

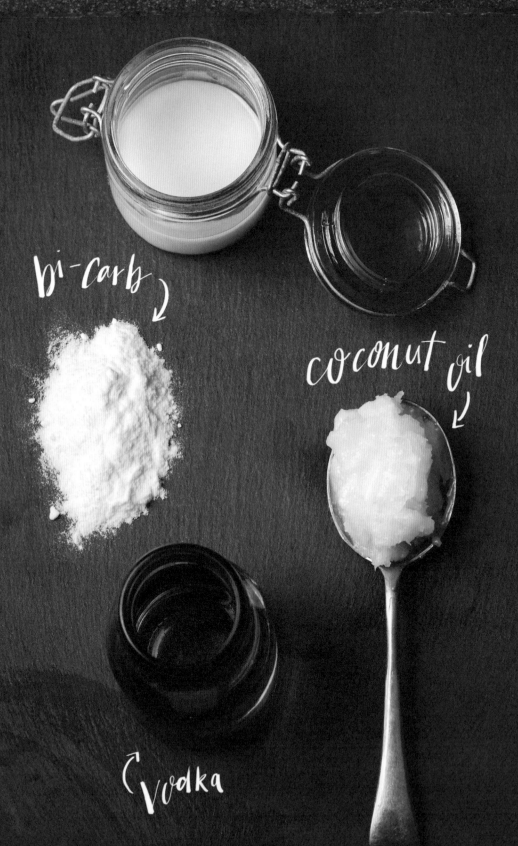

bi-carb

coconut oil

vodka

So what is a *gua sha*?

The BEST thing about a *gua sha* is that you can make it at home with ingredients you probably already have in your pantry . . . in less than 30 seconds!

All you need is vodka (make sure it's triple distilled), aluminum-free bi-carb soda, coconut oil and a jar with a lid.

Fill about 80 per cent of the jar with the bi-carb soda. Add the vodka to the top of the bi-carb, let it absorb through and mix until it has a putty consistency.

Get into the shower and wet your body. Turn the water off and apply the *gua sha* mixture all over your body, avoiding private parts – trust me, sister, those areas and vodka do not mix well together. Eeeek, haha.

Once the *gua sha* is applied, get a loofah or body glove and rub in circular motions all over your body. It might tingle a little bit but don't worry!

Once you have exfoliated your entire body, continue showering as you usually would. Make sure you wash off all of the *gua sha*.

Towel dry before applying coconut oil from head to toe. Your skin will absorb all of the oil and will feel heavenly and supple for days.

I do this two or three times each week for amazing, glowing, healthy skin.

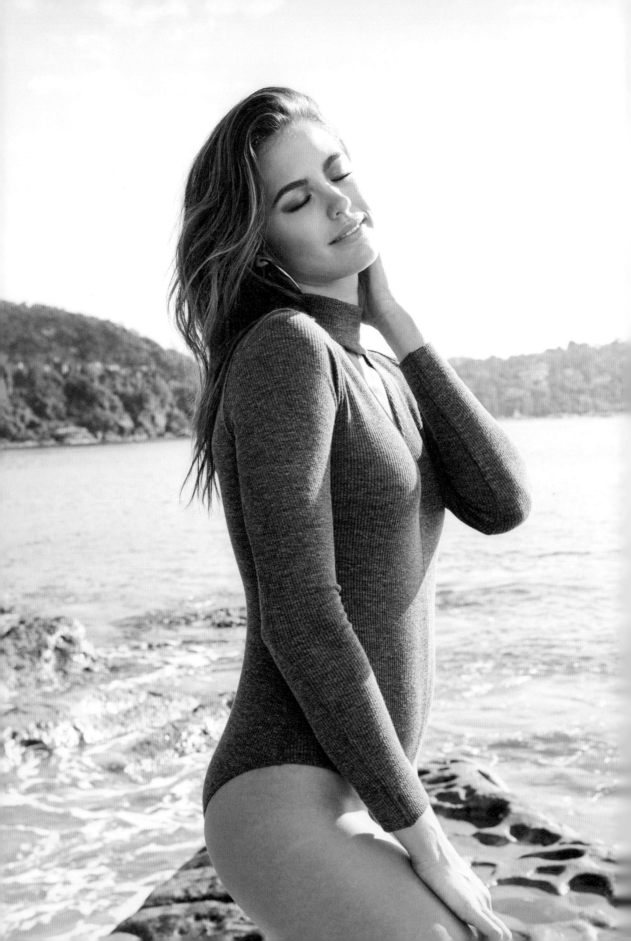

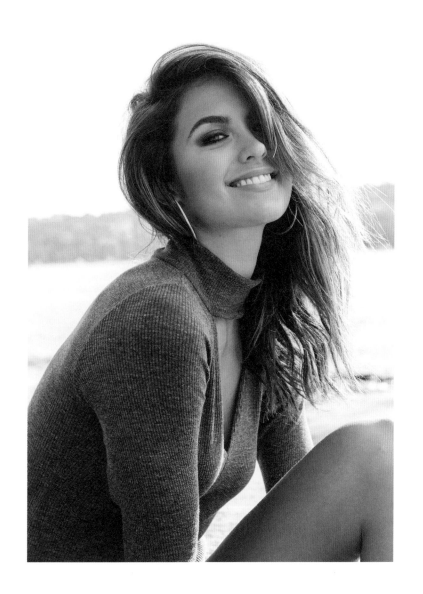

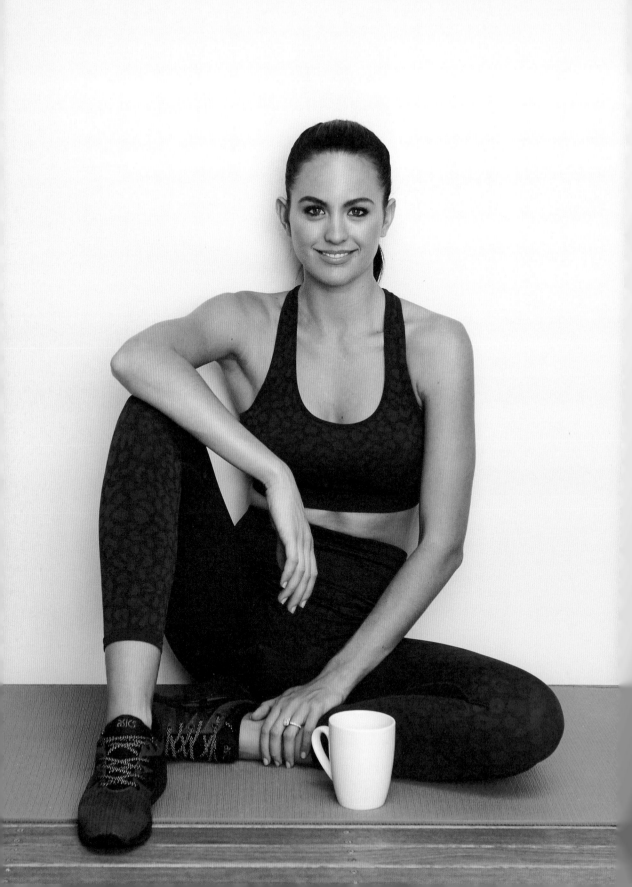

Exercise

My top 5 exercises

THESE ARE MY TOP 5 go-to exercises. I can create a workout using any of these movements, no matter where I am in the world, and I don't need a gym or any equipment to complete them, which means there are zero excuses.

Lunges

Lunges are a dynamic movement that your legs and bum can really benefit from! You can do them in a reverse or forward movement, you can add weights if you are in the gym, and you can even do jump lunges, which raise your heart rate and create a great cardiovascular workout that will make you sweat.

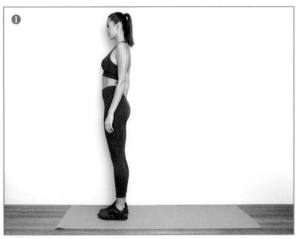
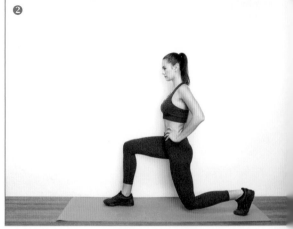

Squats

I refer to these as 'the booty builders'. Squatting is such a great foundation on which you can build an entire workout. If you do enough of these, you will see your butt completely change shape and lift! Just like lunges, you can make squats as challenging as you wish; try jump squats, adding weights, and squat holds on or off a wall.

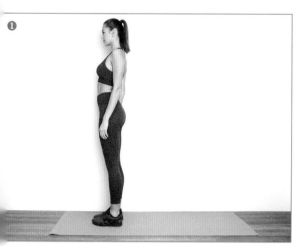

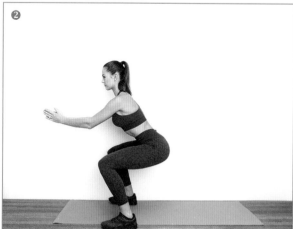

Planks

I get asked a lot how I keep my arms toned; I enjoy boxing and regularly do weights, and I love planking. If you engage your core properly, your arms and abs get a workout so it's a 2-in-1 exercise!

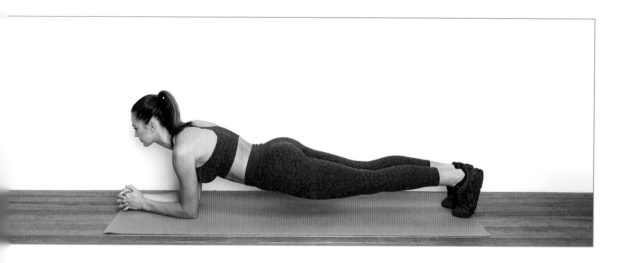

Burpees

I have a massive love-hate relationship with burpees but they are such great cardio and overall body workers that I can't leave them out of my top 5. If I don't have time to get out and go for a run when I'm travelling and there is no gym available, then I will do these in my hotel room along with some lunges, squats and a quick little ab routine (see my Ab workouts on page 85).

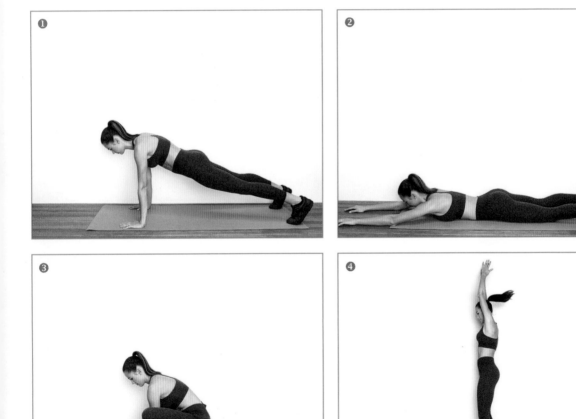

Sit-ups

These are so great for your core and very efficient if you do them properly! If time allows, I will often end my workouts with some core exercises – sit-ups are usually my first choice.

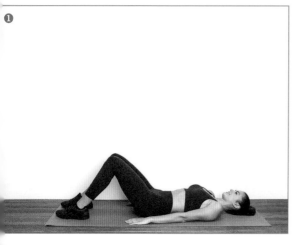

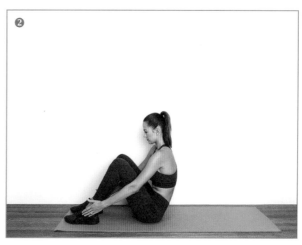

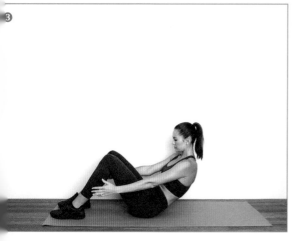

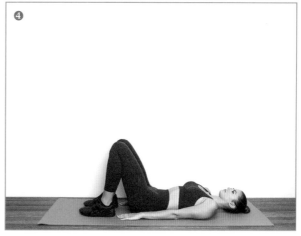

4-week training program

HERE IS A TRAINING program that my personal trainer, Dan Adair, put together for me. I do this in the lead-up to a big swimwear shoot or show and find that it really helps me feel fitter and more toned. I constantly set new goals and change up my training program so that I'm always improving and don't get bored doing the same old thing day in and day out. I have tailored this program to suit a person with medium fitness, but anyone can do this. If you stick diligently to the 4-week program, eat healthy and drink lots of water, you will feel and see the difference. For this training program to work most effectively, stick to these golden rules:

1. Do not miss a workout. Schedule your training into your calendar as you would a business meeting or appointment, or do it with a friend or your partner and hold each other accountable.

2. Cut out or cut back on the amount of sugar you consume.

3. Drink 1–3 litres of water per day. Carry around a bottle of water with you. Make it a habit.

4. NO alcohol. Don't get me wrong, I love a glass of wine, but when you're trying to get fit and healthy, alcohol will set you back 10 steps. It's only 4 weeks; you won't regret it.

WEEK 1

Go hard on day one! ✓

MONDAY	50 bum lifts		**THURSDAY**	Rest Day

MONDAY
50 bum lifts
50 reverse lunges
1km bike ride
40 reverse lunges
40 deep squats
2km bike ride
30 bum lifts
30 deep squats
3km bike ride
20 reverse lunges
20 deep squats
4km bike ride
10 reverse lunges
10 deep squats
5km bike ride

TUESDAY
1 hour power walk OR
3–5km run
Ab workout #1

(or select from workouts
1–4, see page 85)

WEDNESDAY
Complete 10 rounds of:
1 minute row (I aim for
250m per minute,
but do what feels
comfortable
for you)
2 minutes rest
6 squat jumps

THURSDAY
Rest Day

FRIDAY
Complete 5 rounds of:
10 deep squats with
weights
10 burpees
1 minute rest

Complete 5 rounds of:
10 lunges
10 burpees
1 minute rest

Complete 5 rounds of:
10 kettlebell swings
10 burpees
1 minute rest

SATURDAY
Walk for 45 minutes –
1 hour
Ab workout #2

(or select from workouts
1–4, see page 85)

SUNDAY
Rest Day

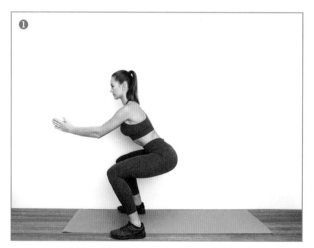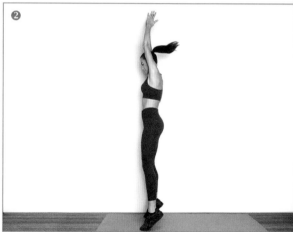

SQUAT JUMP

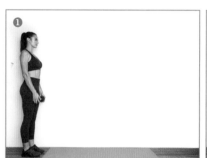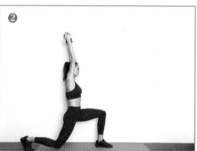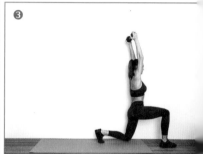

WALKING LUNGE

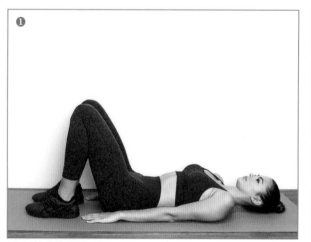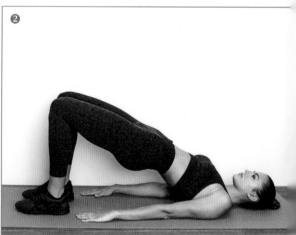

BUM LIFT

WEEK 2

MONDAY	50 bum lifts
	50 reverse lunges
	1km bike ride
	40 reverse lunges
	40 deep squats
	2km bike ride
	30 bum lifts
	30 deep squats
	3km bike ride
	20 reverse lunges
	20 deep squats
	4km bike ride
	10 reverse lunges
	10 deep squats
	5km bike ride

TUESDAY	1 hour power walk OR
	3–5km run
	Ab workout #3
	(or select from workouts
	1–4, see page 85)

WEDNESDAY	Complete 15 rounds of:
	200m sprint
	200m walk

THURSDAY	1 hour power walk OR
	3–5km run
	Ab workout #4
	(or select from workouts
	1–4, see page 85)

FRIDAY	Complete 10 rounds of:
	10 walking lunges
	10 squat jumps
	10 medicine ball slams
	100m row
	2 minutes rest

SATURDAY	Walk for 45 minutes –
	1 hour
	Ab workout #1
	(or select from workouts
	1–4, see page 85)

SUNDAY	Rest Day

WEEK 3

For the exercises using weights this week, choose a weight that is comfortable for you, usually between 4–8 kg.

MONDAY

Complete 4 rounds of:
10 deep squats with weights
10 lunge jumps with weights
500m ride (set to level 10, complete in under 50 seconds)
1 minute rest

Complete 4 rounds of:
16 reverse lunges with weights
10 squat jumps with weights
200m cross trainer (set to level 12, complete in under 60 seconds)

TUESDAY

1 hour power walk OR
    3–5km run
Ab workout #2

(or select from workouts
    1–4, see page 85)

WEDNESDAY

Complete 20 rounds of:
200m sprint
200m walk

THURSDAY

Rest Day

FRIDAY

Complete 10 rounds of:
1 minute row
2 minutes rest
10 squat jumps

SATURDAY

Walk for 45 minutes –
    1 hour
Ab workout #3

(or select from workouts
    1–4, see page 85)

SUNDAY

Rest Day

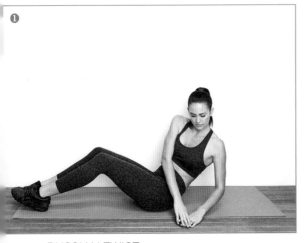 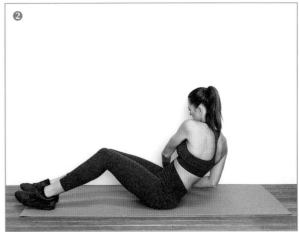

RUSSIAN TWIST

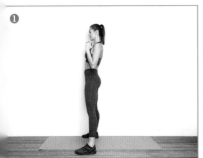 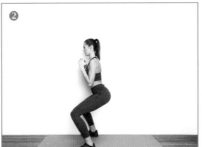 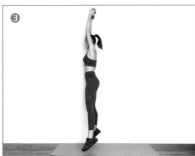

SQUAT JUMP WITH WEIGHTS

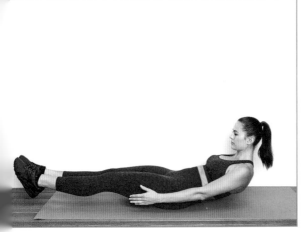

REVERSE PLANK

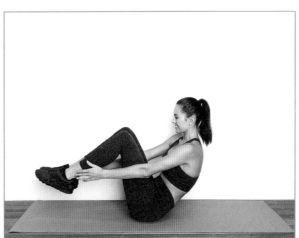

V SIT

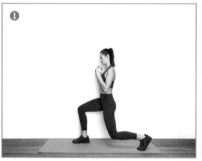 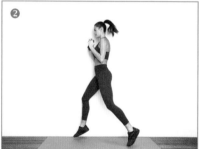 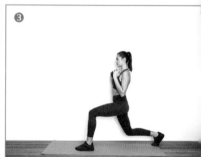

LUNGE JUMP WITH WEIGHTS

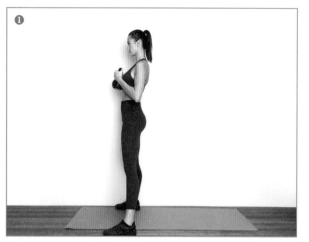 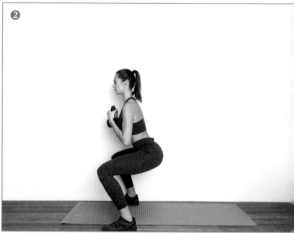

DEEP SQUAT WITH WEIGHTS

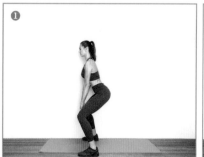 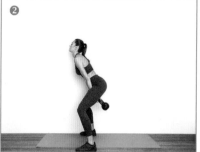 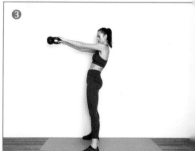

KETTLEBELL SWING

WEEK 4

MONDAY — Complete 5 rounds of:
20 walking lunges (I use a 5–10kg plate)
15–20 burpees
500m ride (set to level 10, complete in under 50 seconds)
2 minutes rest

Complete 10 rounds of:
1 kettlebell swing with a 30 second prone hold in between each set
15–30 seconds rest

TUESDAY — 5km run
Ab workout #4

(or select from workouts 1–4, see page 85)

WEDNESDAY — Complete 6 rounds of:
1000m treadmill sprints

THURSDAY — Rest Day

FRIDAY — Complete 5 rounds of:
10 deep squats with weights
10 burpees
1 minute rest

Complete 5 rounds of:
10 kettlebell swings
10 burpees
1 minute rest

SATURDAY — Complete 10 rounds of:
1 minute row (aim for 250m per minute)
2 minutes rest
10 jump squats

SUNDAY — Rest Day

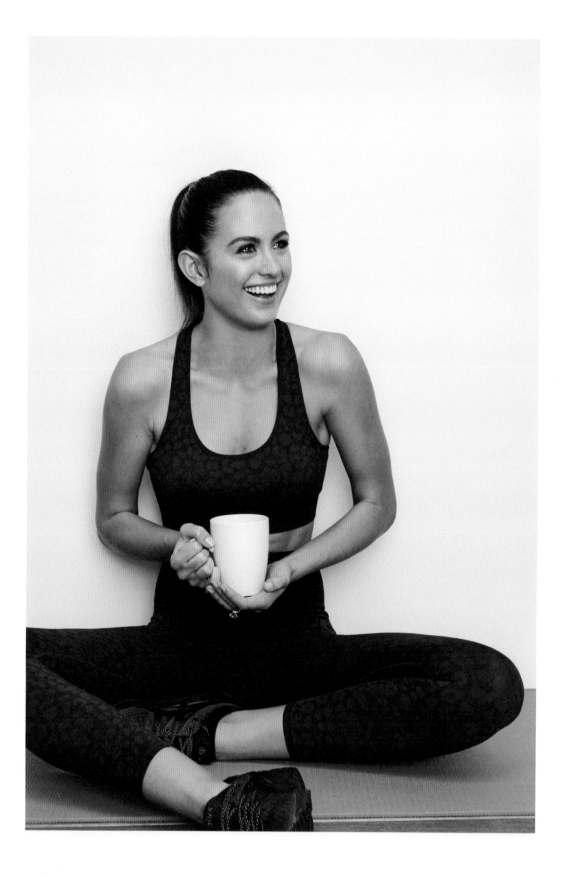

AB WORKOUTS

Feel free to switch between Ab workouts during your 4-week plan. Changing it up can keep it exciting and it's important to always push yourself!

AB WORKOUT 1	**Complete 5 rounds of:** 20 sit-ups 30 second – 1 minute reverse plank/prone hold

AB WORKOUT 2	**Complete 5 rounds of:** 20 sit-ups 20 medicine ball slams

AB WORKOUT 3	**Complete 5 rounds of:** 20 V sits 20 Russian twists 30 second plank

AB WORKOUT 4	**Complete 3 rounds of:** 25 sit-ups 25 V sits 25 crunches 25 Russian twists

Good luck!

I believe in you! Make sure you tag me in your pics on social media and let me know how you're going with your #JC4Weekchallenge.

Recipes

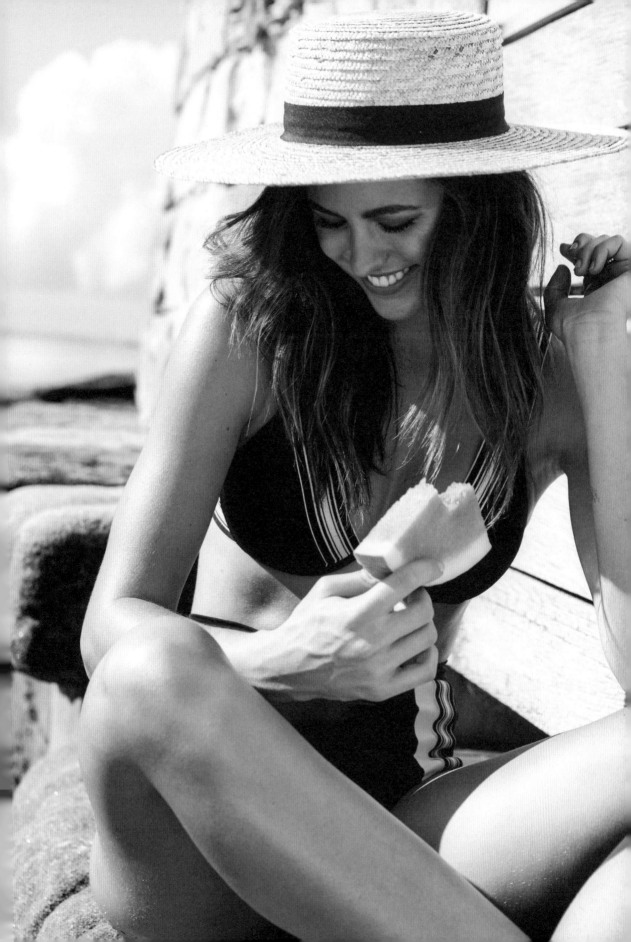

Food for a healthy body and life

BEING HEALTHY SHOULDN'T BE hard and it shouldn't take up lots of your time to prepare nutritious meals. A lot of us are time poor, we work hard and have lots of things on our plate (pun unintended). The fact we don't have much spare time does not mean our health should be compromised, which is why I have put together my favourite recipes for you. They are easy to make and won't take too long to prepare. This is what I eat, it's what fuels my body and keeps me energised throughout the day. I hope you enjoy these meals and they make you feel healthy and full of life!

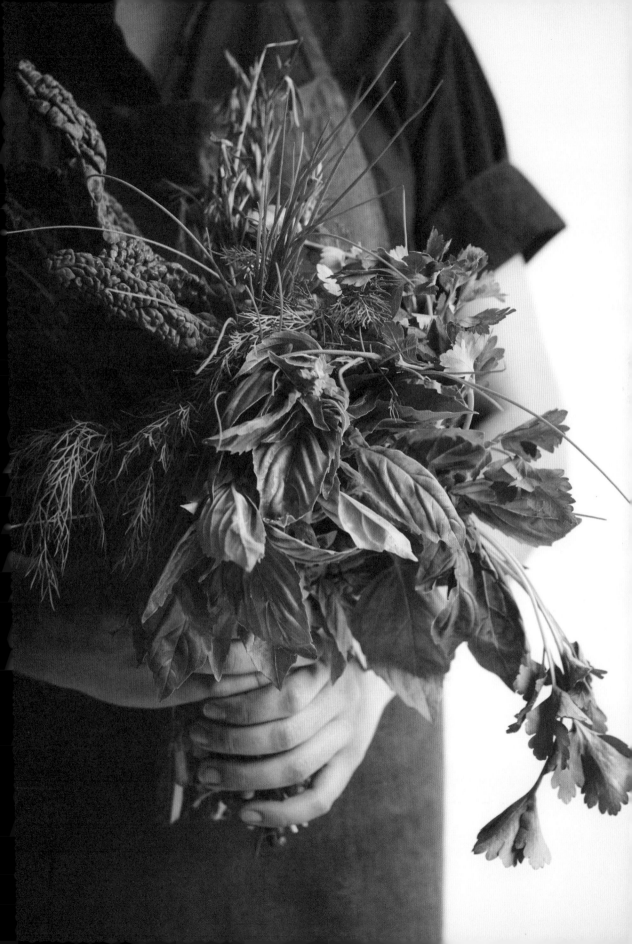

Tofu

Dark Chocolate

Almond Milk

Eggs

Chicken

Coconut
Water

Dates

Tamari

Goat's
Feta

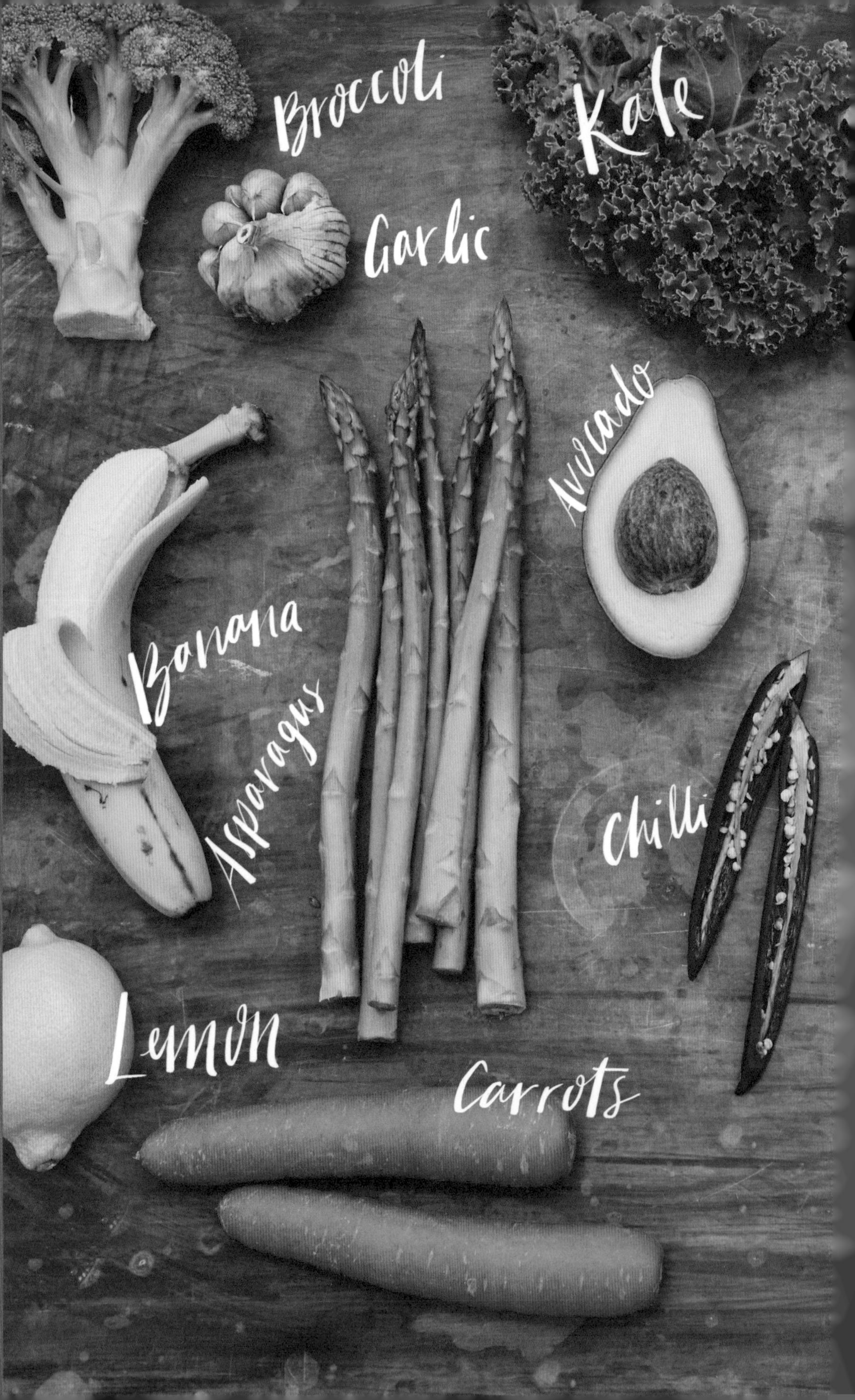

Broccoli

Kale

Garlic

Avocado

Banana

Asparagus

Chilli

Lemon

Carrots

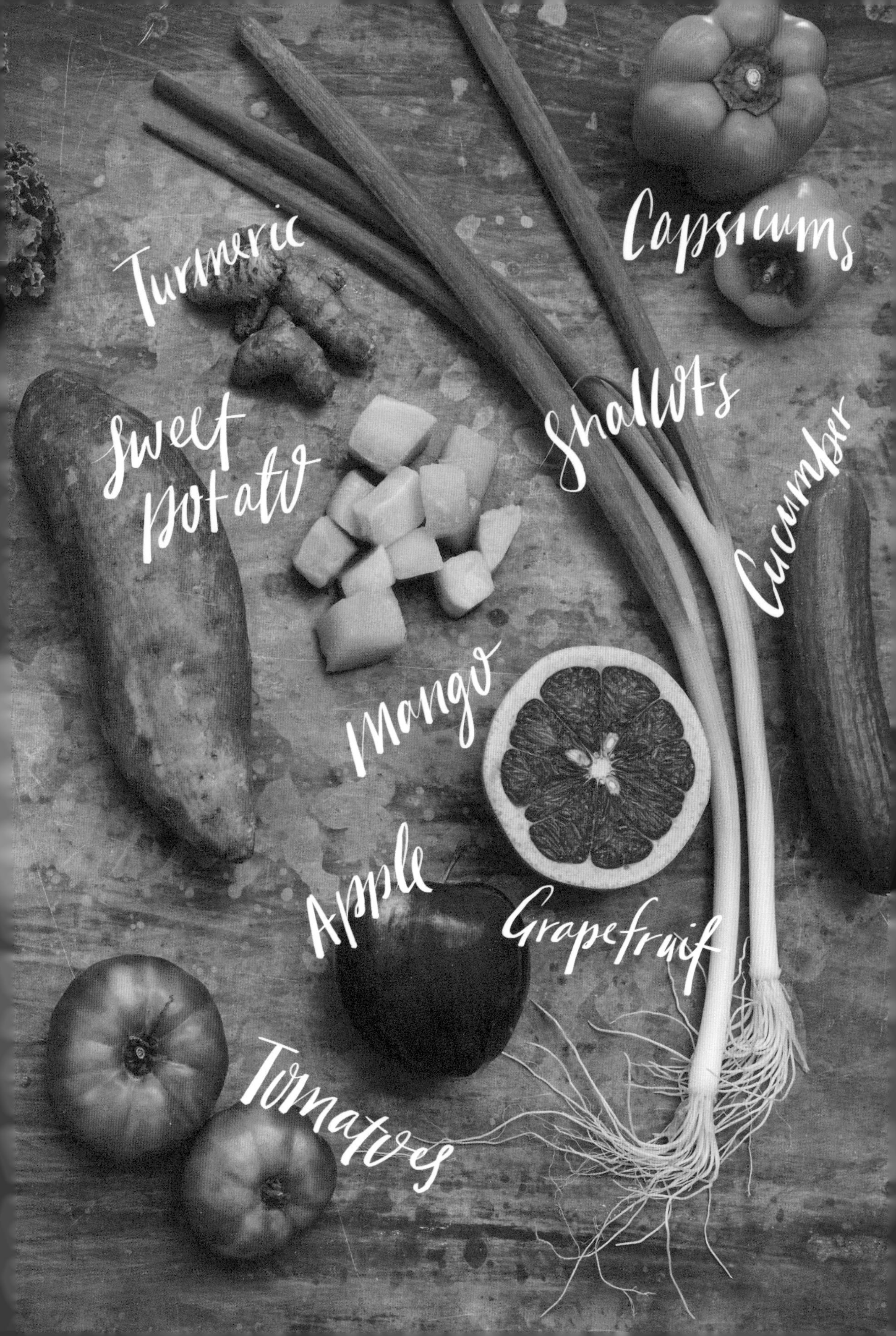

Turmeric

Capsicums

Sweet Potato

Shallots

Cucumber

Mango

Grapefruit

Apple

Tomatoes

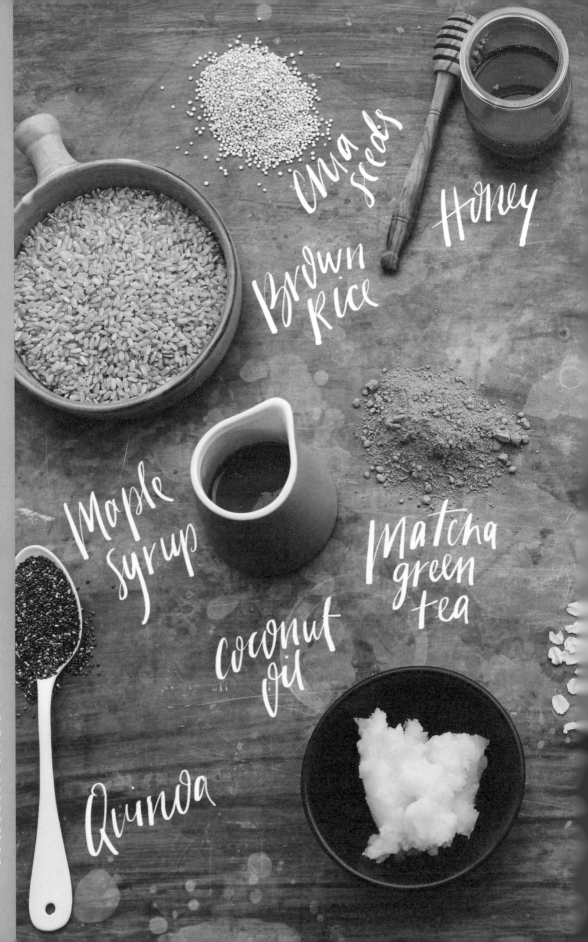

Chia seeds

Honey

Brown Rice

Maple Syrup

Matcha green tea

coconut Oil

Quinoa

pepper

pink
sea
salt

olive oil

pepitas

oats

coconut
milk

Almonds

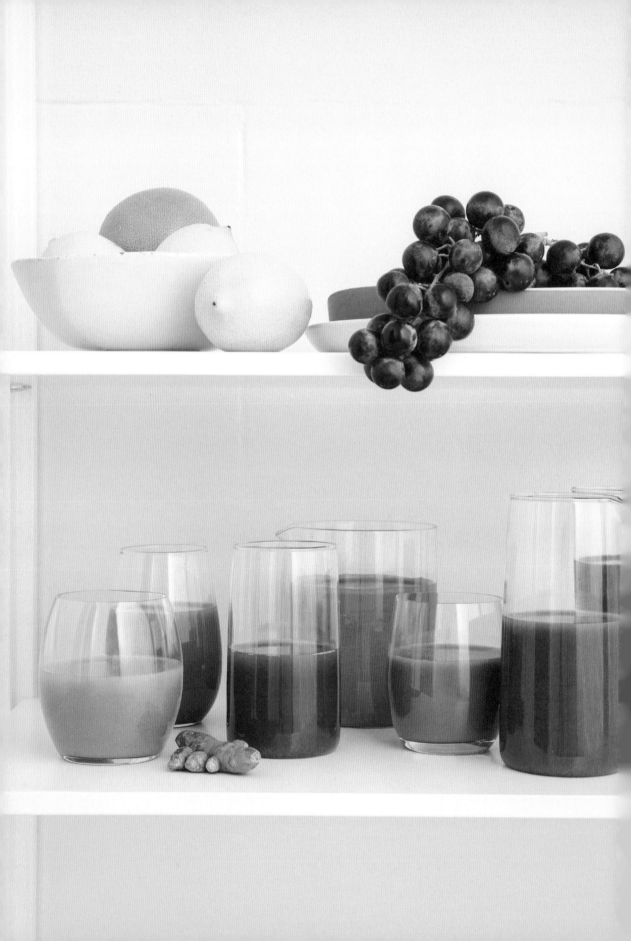

juices, smoothies & snacks

Healing Turmeric Juice

My go-to juice when I feel a cold coming on.

Ingredients

2 apples

1 lemon, skin removed

2 carrots

2 × 2cm pieces fresh ginger

2 × 2cm pieces fresh turmeric, peeled

handful ice

pinch of black pepper

Chop the apples, lemon and carrots into juicing-sized pieces. Put all the ingredients through the juicer.

Pour into a glass, stir in some ice to chill and add a pinch of pepper.

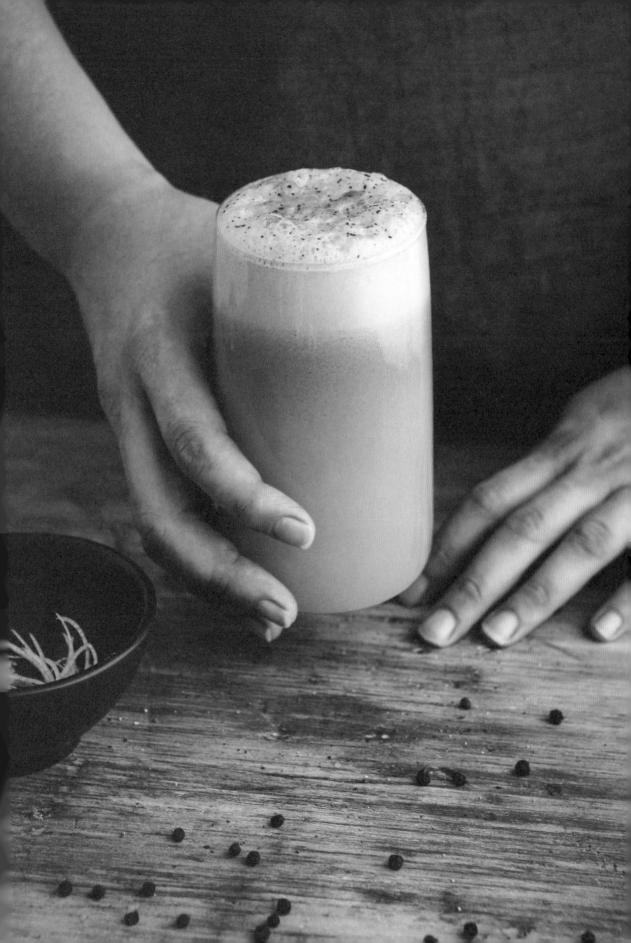

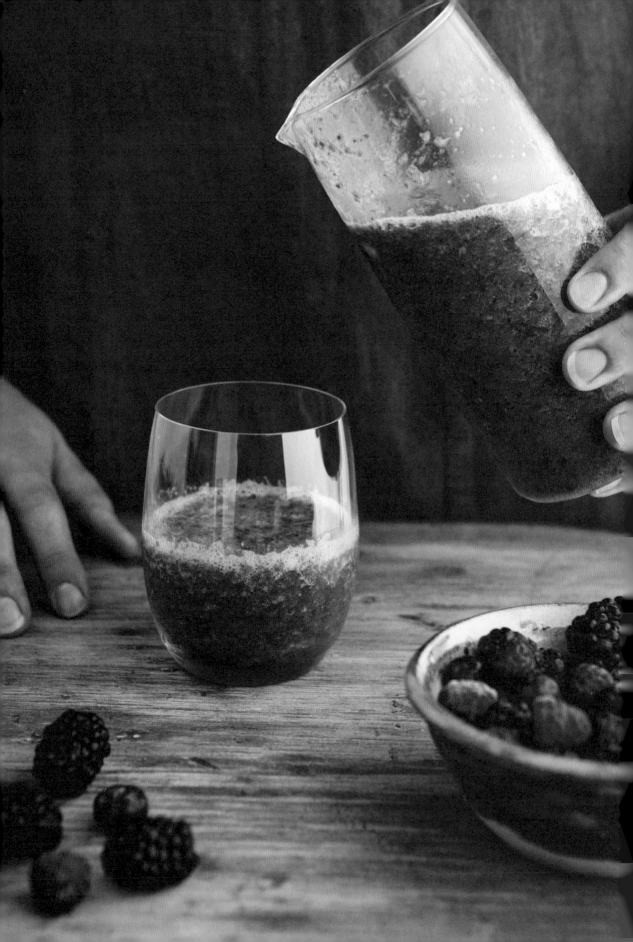

Berry Energiser

Quick 'n' easy, I love this before a workout. It gives me the energy boost I need before exercising.

Ingredients

½ cup frozen berries (mixed, or I love raspberries)

½ cup frozen banana

handful baby spinach leaves

1 cup cold water

Put the berries, banana and spinach through a juicer or blender, adding the cold water as needed to get the consistency you like.

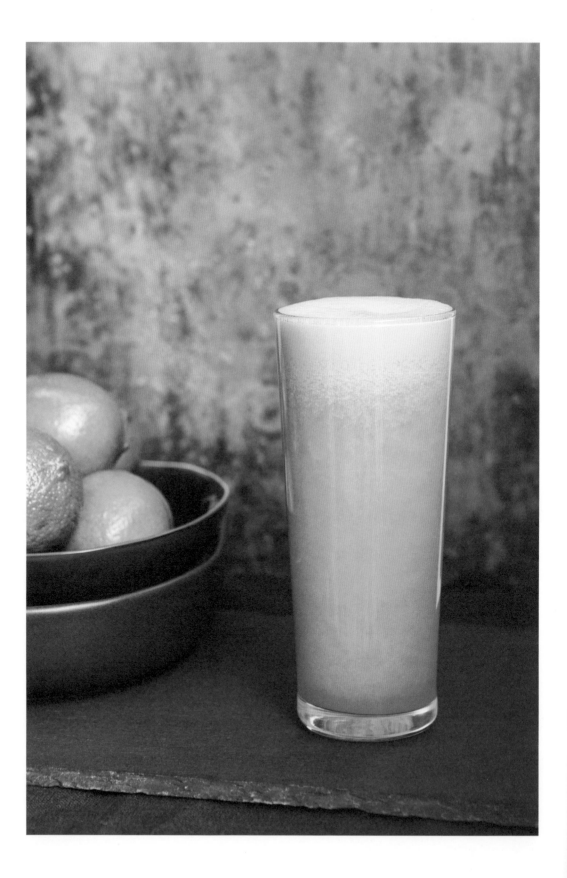

Zingy Pineapple Juice

The ultimate summer juice!

Ingredients

½ pineapple, peeled

2cm piece fresh ginger

1 lime, skin removed

½ long red chilli, or to taste

Chop all the ingredients into juicing-sized pieces and feed through a juicer or blender. Add chilli to taste.

The Green Goddess

This smoothie has an abundance of goodness that makes you feel so full of life!

Ingredients

½ mango, skin removed

½ lemon, skin removed

handful baby spinach leaves

1 medjool date, pit removed

1 teaspoon chia seeds

½ cup cold water

Chop the mango and lemon into juicing-sized pieces. Put all the ingredients through a juicer or blender, adding cold water as needed.

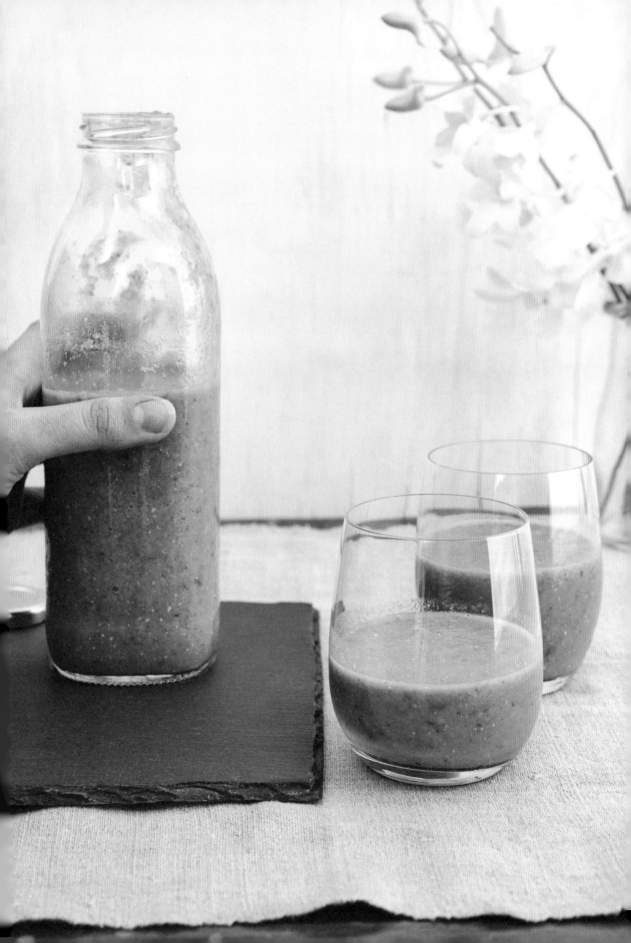

Green Power Boost

Packed full of nutrients, I always make this smoothie if I have an early start on set. I drink it during hair and makeup prep.

Ingredients

½ orange, skin removed

½ banana, peeled

big handful baby spinach leaves

1 medjool date, pit removed

½ teaspoon spirulina

1 teaspoon chia seeds

Chop the orange and banana into juicing-sized pieces. Put all the ingredients through a juicer or blender. Add one or two tablespoons of water to reach your desired consistency.

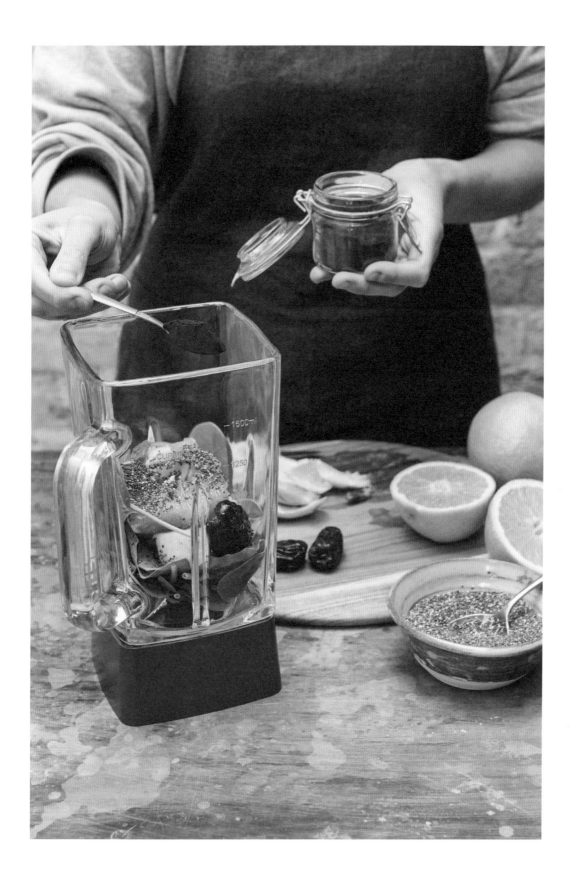

Choc Smoothie

This is my Aunty Cynthia's recipe and it's my ultimate arvo pick-me-up. Whenever I have this I think of her and all our wonderful cooking memories!

Ingredients

½ cup raw cashews

2 medjool dates, pits removed

2–3 tablespoons raw cacao powder

3 handfuls ice

pinch of pink sea salt

2 tablespoons cacao nibs

Put all the ingredients in a blender and blitz until you reach your desired consistency.

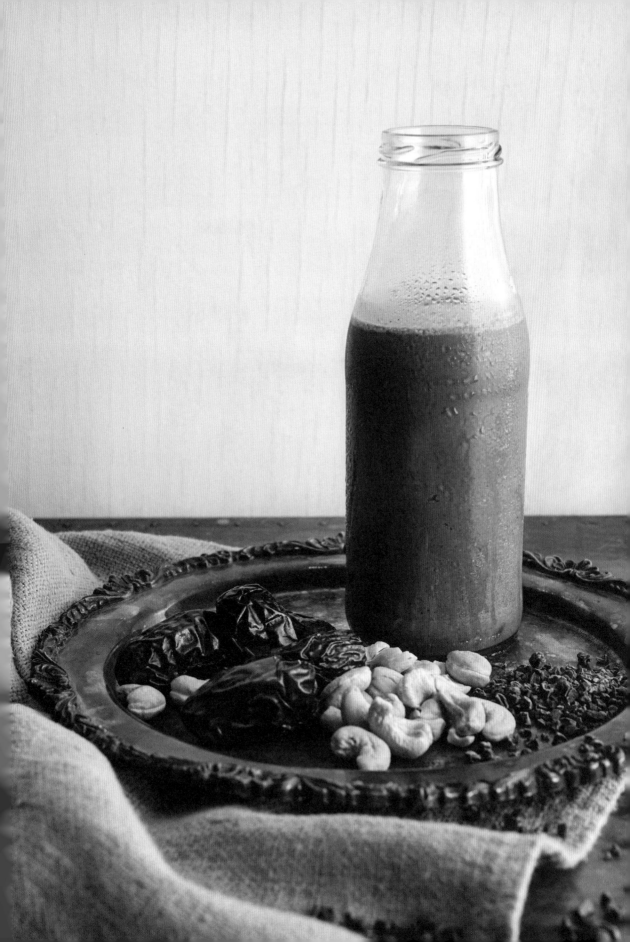

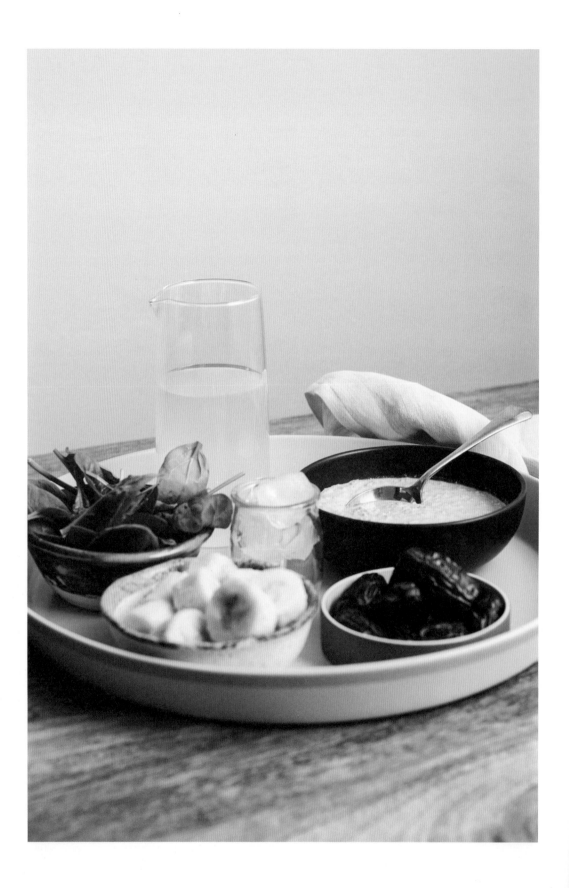

Brekky Smoothie

A meal in a smoothie!

Ingredients

1 cup oats, soaked overnight
   in water

1 frozen banana, chopped

1 cup baby spinach leaves

2 medjool dates, pits removed

1 cup coconut water

handful ice

Put all the ingredients in a blender and blitz until you reach your desired consistency.

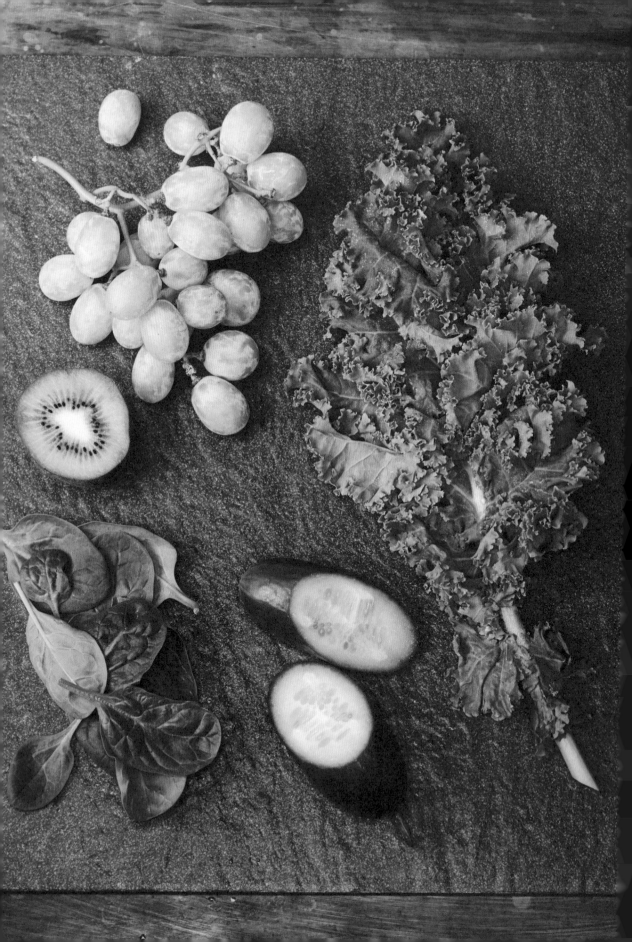

Alkalising Green Smoothie

Whenever my skin starts breaking out, I drink one of these with every meal. In two days I notice a difference.

Ingredients

1 small bunch kale

1 Lebanese cucumber

1 kiwifruit, peeled

handful baby spinach leaves

¾ cup green grapes

Roughly chop the kale, cucumber and kiwifruit into blender-sized pieces. Place all the ingredients in a blender and blitz until smooth.

Sunshine Smoothie

This summery smoothie reminds me of being on a romantic holiday in Bora Bora. Good times!

Ingredients

½ lime (skin on)

1 frozen banana, peeled

1 cup diced fresh pineapple

handful ice

½ cup water

Cut the lime and banana into blender-sized pieces. Put all the ingredients in a blender and blitz until you reach your desired consistency.

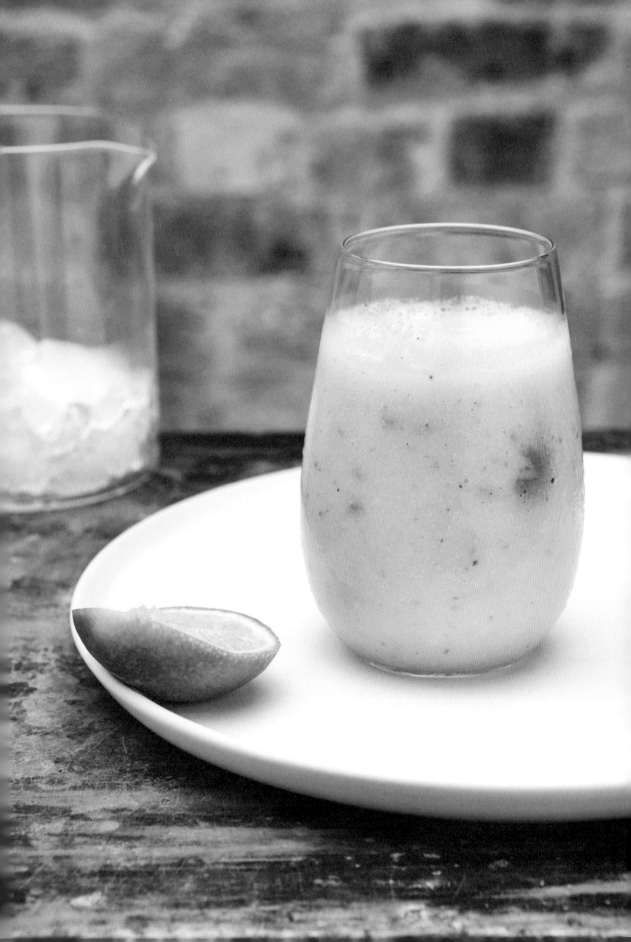

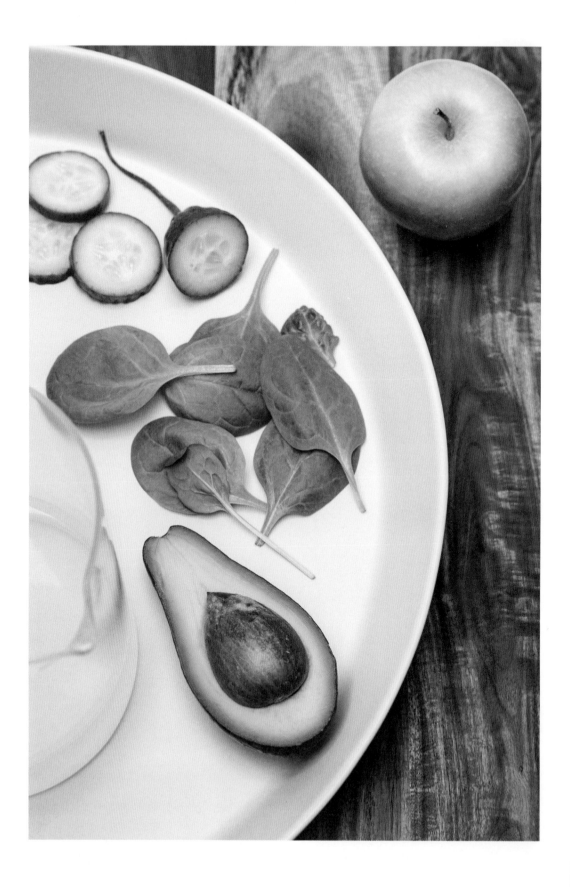

Skin-loving Smoothie

The omegas found in the avo will make you glow from the inside out.

Ingredients

1 medium cucumber

1 large green apple

½ avocado

2 cups baby spinach leaves

½ cup coconut water

Roughly chop the cucumber into blender-sized pieces. Remove the core from the apple, keeping the skin on, then chop the apple into pieces. Place the remaining ingredients in a blender and blitz until smooth.

Nut Milks

Nut milks are super easy and quick to make. They are amazing in smoothies, with your muesli or simply enjoyed on their own. I usually only use cashews, hazelnuts or almonds; this is just personal preference, though. My Aunty Cynthia taught me how to make nut milks. A golden lesson I'll never forget!

Ingredients

1 cup raw nuts of your choice

pinch of pink sea salt

3–4 cups water, filtered preferred

Make sure you soak the nuts overnight, between 8 and 12 hours is ideal. Drain soaking water and rinse the nuts well.

Place in a Vitamix or high-powered blender with salt and 3 cups water – if you don't want your milk too thick or creamy, add another cup of water. Blend for about 1 minute or until the consistency is smooth.

To remove the nut pulp from the liquid, strain through a muslin/cheesecloth – if you can't get one from your local health food store, you can use a clean stocking.

Pour the strained milk into an airtight jar and there you have your nut milk! Keep in the fridge for up to 1 week.

TIP: FOR SOMETHING DIFFERENT, ADD VANILLA BEAN SEEDS OR CINNAMON TO YOUR MIX. IT'S SUPER DELICIOUS AND MAKES FOR A NICE AFTERNOON SNACK WITH A PROTEIN BALL (SEE PEANUT BUTTER ENERGY BALLS ON PAGE 127 AND GINGER & DATE POWERBALLS ON PAGE 129).

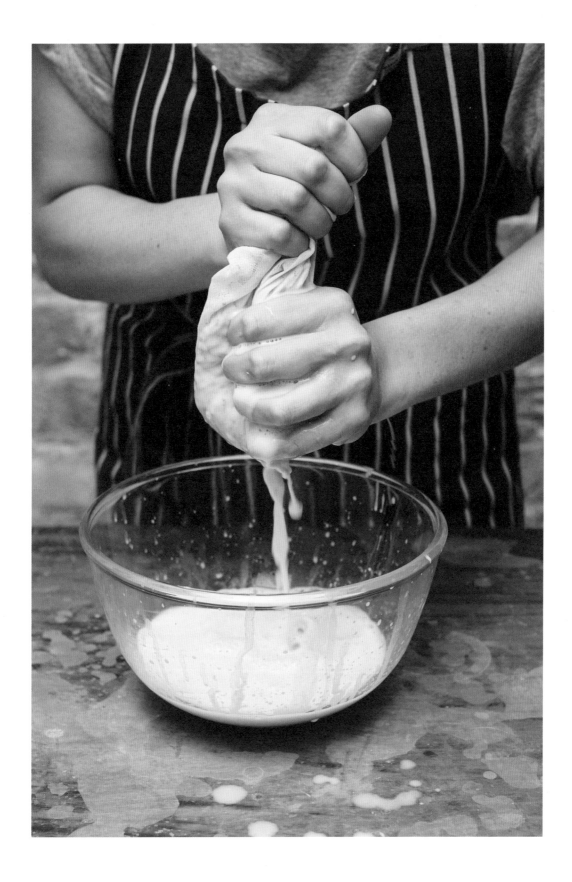

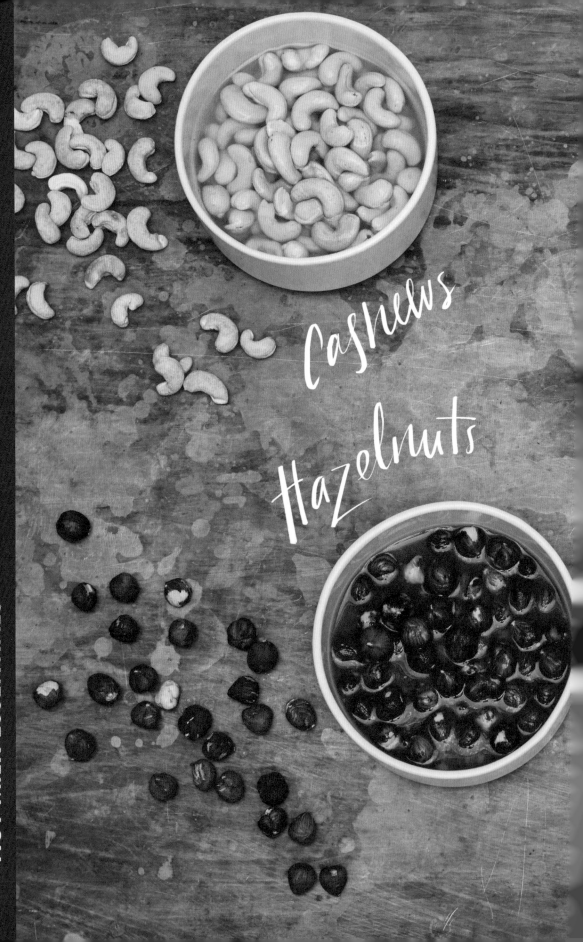

Cashews

Hazelnuts

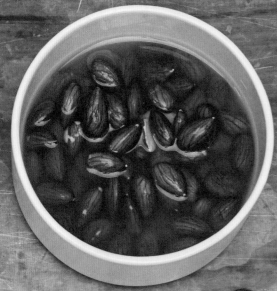

Almonds

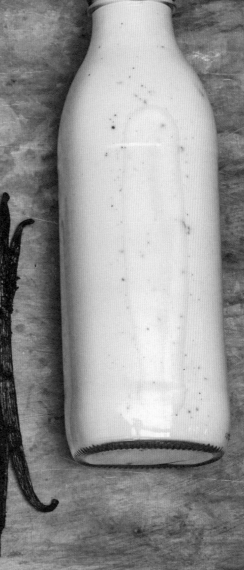

Cinnamon

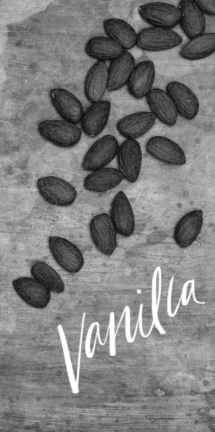

Vanilla

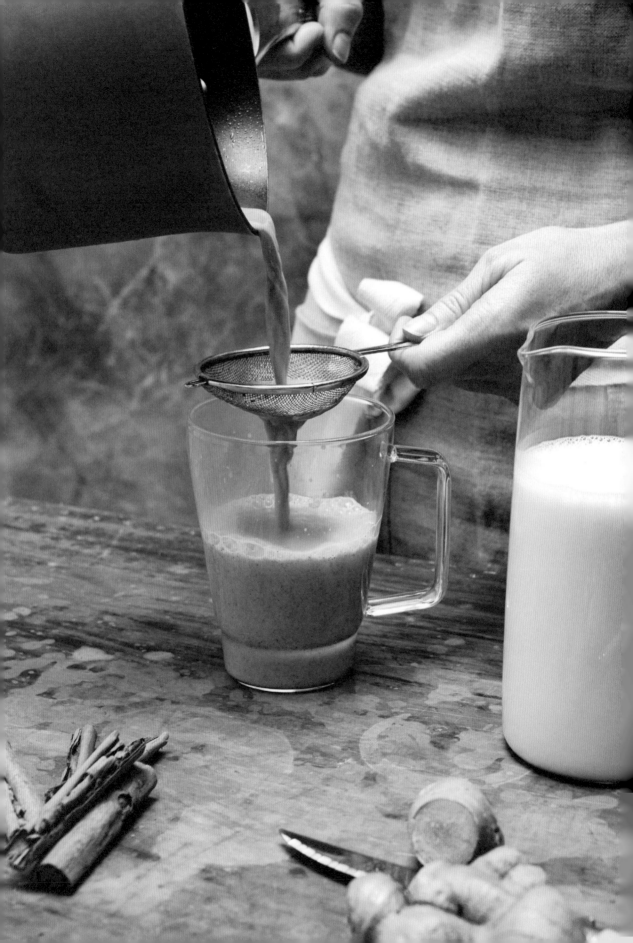

Warming Ginger Nut Milk

A magical winter warmer . . . an after-dinner delight.
Just add an open fire and you have the perfect night.

Ingredients

1½ cups nut milk of your choice
(see page 118)

3cm piece fresh ginger, peeled

1 teaspoon cinnamon

In a small saucepan, bring the nut milk to a light simmer over a very low heat. Finely grate the ginger and add to the milk with the cinnamon. Allow to heat gently for about 5 minutes so the spice can infuse the milk. Don't let the mix boil. Strain and serve in a mug on a cold day.

If you want your milk extra zingy, add more ginger.

Snack Seed Bars

A bar of this, a peppermint tea and a good book – the ideal afternoon.

Ingredients

250g pitted medjool dates, roughly chopped

2 teaspoons cinnamon

1 cup almonds, roughly chopped

1 cup walnuts, roughly chopped

½ cup pumpkin seeds

½ cup flaxseeds

½ cup chia seeds

Preheat the oven to 180°C. Line a small square baking tin (about 20 × 20cm) with baking paper.

In a saucepan over medium heat, place the dates, cinnamon and about 1½ cups water. Bring this to a gentle simmer for about 6 minutes. Transfer the hot mixture to your blender, or use a stick blender, and blitz to a smooth consistency.

Place remaining ingredients in a large bowl, add the date puree and mix with a wooden spoon until well combined. Pour the mix into your prepared tin and use your wooden spoon to even out the top and spread right into the corners. For extra crunch, add some roughly chopped almonds, pumpkin seeds and flaxseeds on top.

Bake for about 20–25 minutes until browned on top but not too crisp!

Allow to cool in the tin before cutting into 12 rectangular bars. These will keep in an airtight container in the fridge for about a week.

Makes 12

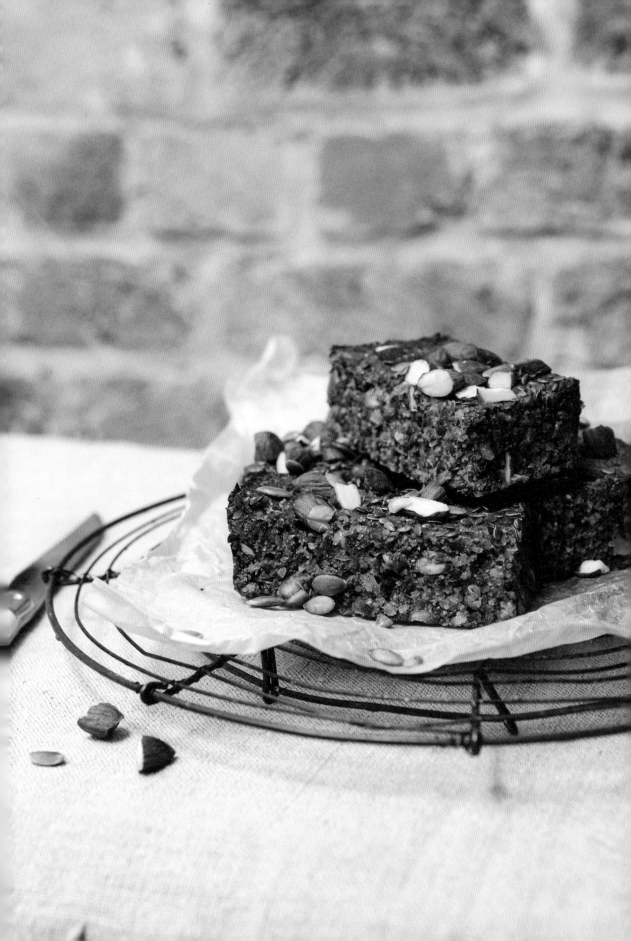

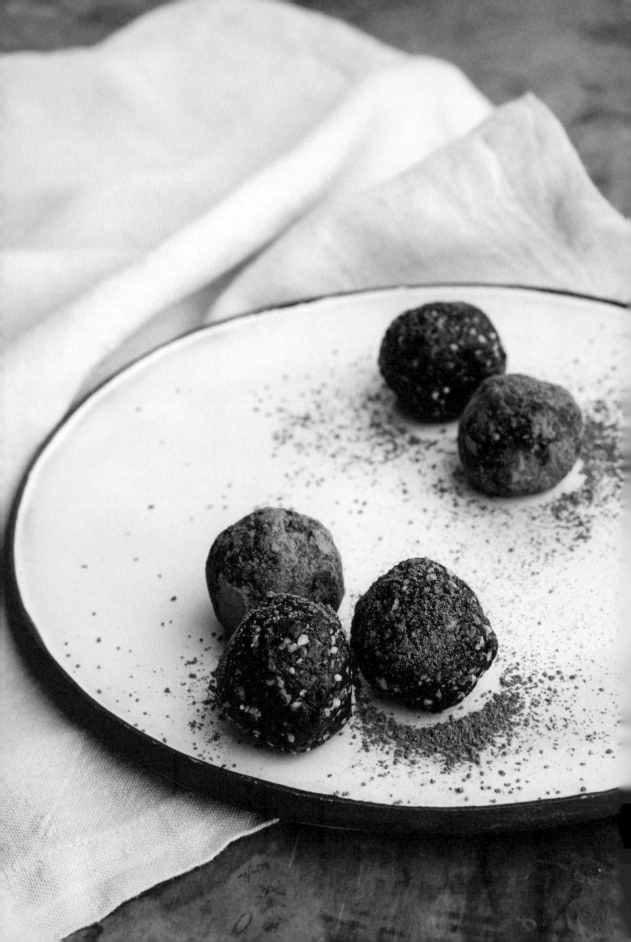

Peanut Butter Energy Balls

If I am working out in the afternoon, I enjoy one (or two) of these while I drive to the gym!

Ingredients

1 cup raw almonds

200g pitted medjool dates

2 tablespoons natural peanut butter

2 tablespoons raw cacao

Place all the ingredients in the bowl of a food processor or blender and blend until the mix is well combined and there are no large chunks of nuts or dates. Scoop the mix out into a large bowl.

Using your hands (you might like to wear gloves for this part), roll the mix into balls roughly 2–3cm in size and place them in a container lined with baking paper.

These will keep in your fridge in an airtight container for a week or so.

Makes 24 balls

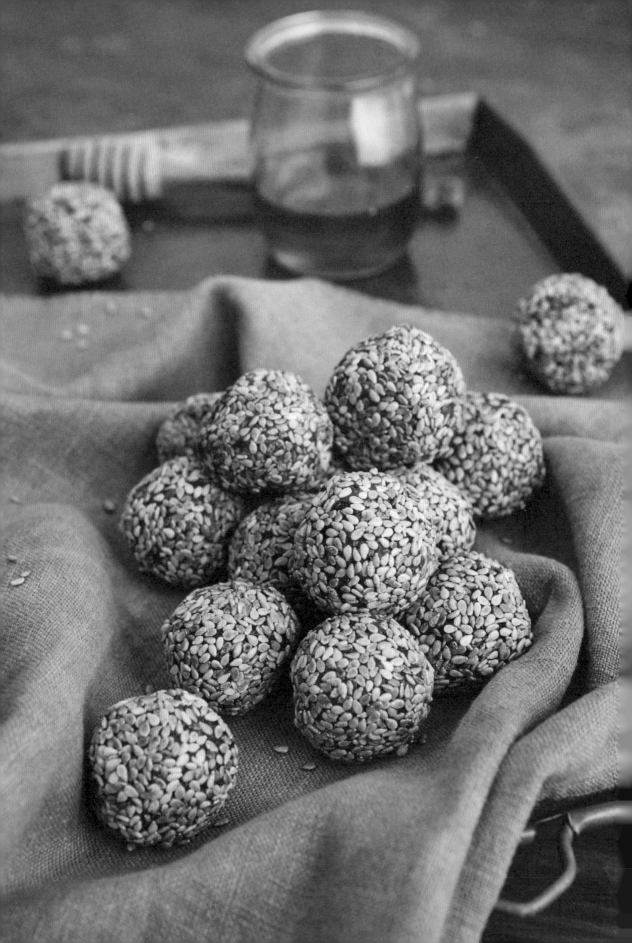

Ginger & Date Powerballs

Powerballs are great for travelling. A few of these on a flight will stop you snacking on anything naughty from the trolley.

Ingredients

1 cup walnuts

250g pitted medjool dates

1 tablespoon honey (I love Manuka honey, but any honey will do)

2cm piece fresh ginger, peeled and finely grated

½ cup toasted sesame seeds

Place the walnuts, dates, honey and ginger in the bowl of a food processor and blend until well combined. There should not be any large chunks of nuts or dates remaining. Transfer the mix to a large bowl.

Using your hands (you might like to wear gloves for this), roll the mixture into balls roughly 3cm in size, then roll them gently in the toasted sesame seeds. Place in a container lined with baking paper.

These should keep in your fridge in an airtight container for about a week.

Makes 24 balls

Matcha Energy Balls

YUM! I go to bed dreaming of these.

Ingredients

½ cup dried figs, stalks removed and soaked overnight in water

1 cup raw almonds

1 tablespoon matcha powder

1 teaspoon cinnamon

100g pitted medjool dates

2 tablespoons tahini

⅓ cup desiccated coconut

Place the figs, almonds, matcha, cinnamon, dates and tahini in the bowl of a food processor and blitz until well combined. Transfer the mix to a large bowl.

Using your hands (you might like to use gloves for this), roll the mix into balls roughly 3cm in size, then roll them gently in the desiccated coconut. Place in a container lined with baking paper.

These should keep in your fridge in an airtight container for about a week.

Makes 24 balls

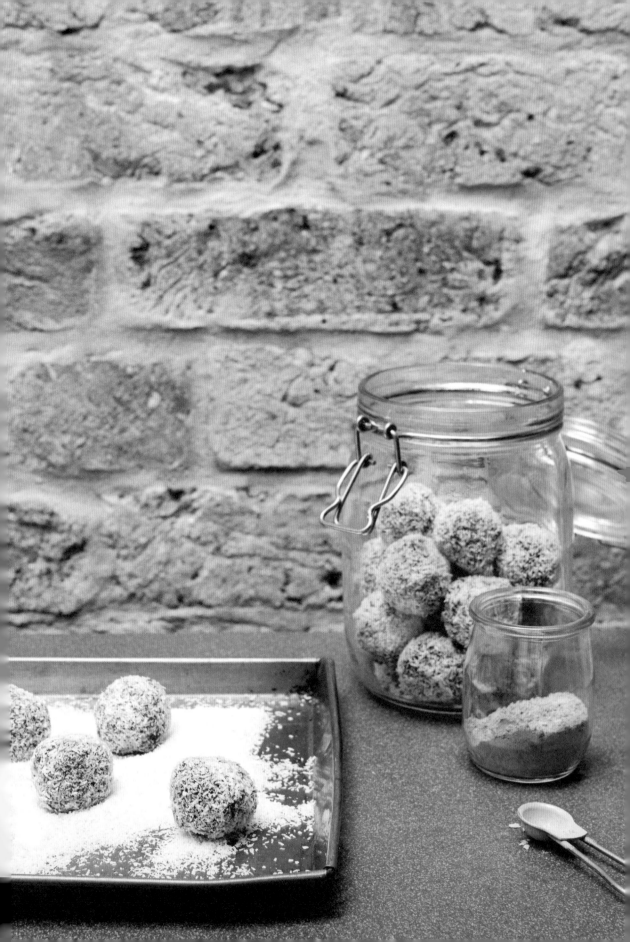

Simple Chicken Broth

Soul food! Broths are incredibly nourishing. A winter staple of mine, this wholesome recipe uses bones left over from a roast chicken, or you can get chicken bones from your butcher. It's even more delicious if you use any leftover broth from the Turmeric Poached Chicken on page 204.

Ingredients

chicken bones, approx. 1.5kg

2–3 stalks celery, roughly chopped

1–2 medium carrots, roughly chopped

1 whole garlic bulb, peeled and smashed

3cm piece fresh ginger, roughly chopped

2cm piece fresh turmeric, roughly chopped

2.5L water (if using leftover broth, add water to make 2.5L total)

15 whole peppercorns

Place all the ingredients in a large stock pot. Bring to a simmer over a low heat then gently simmer for about 2 hours.

Strain the broth to remove and discard the solids. Serve the strained broth warm in a small bowl or mug. Season to taste.

This broth can be frozen in portions and reheated as needed. It will keep for a month or two in an airtight container in your freezer.

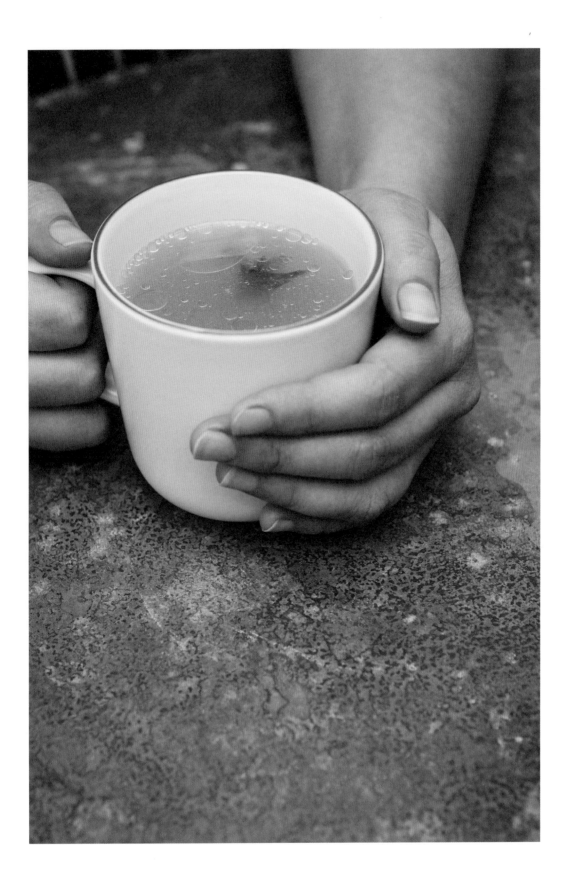

Breakfast

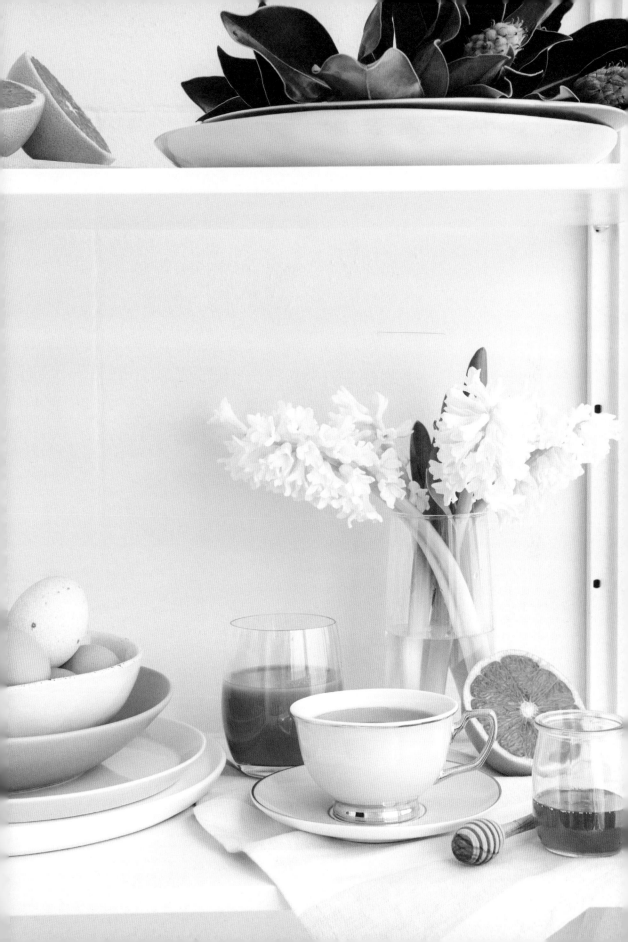

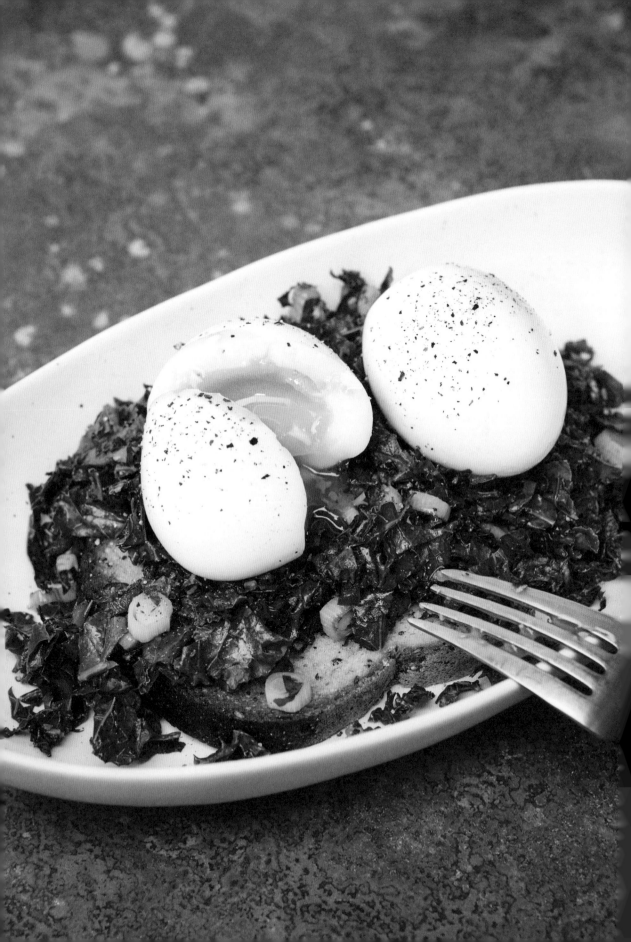

Soft-boiled Eggs with
Kale, Capsicum and Chilli

I never get bored of this brekky! When I'm not travelling or starting work before 5am, I cook this. It sustains me until lunch – I never snack when I have it for breakfast!

Ingredients

olive oil

½ cup diced spring onions

½ cup diced red capsicum

1 teaspoon diced chilli

3 cups finely chopped kale

toast, gluten-free, for serving

2 medium eggs

salt and pepper

Heat the olive oil in a small frying pan over medium heat. Add the spring onions, capsicum and chilli. Sauté until the spring onions are soft. Add the kale and cook until soft.

Bring a saucepan of water to the boil. Add the eggs and leave to cook for 7 minutes. Rinse under cool water and remove shells.

Make your toast then pile it up with the kale mixture, top with the soft-boiled eggs and there you have your brekky.

Serves 1

Breakfast Frittatas

A Sunday fave of mine – I keep one in the fridge and take it to work with me on Monday. My version of a takeaway meal!

Ingredients

6 medium eggs

dash of milk

salt and pepper

120g goat's feta

1 punnet cherry tomatoes, halved

handful baby spinach leaves

1 zucchini, grated

handful fresh basil leaves

handful fresh parsley, finely chopped

Preheat the oven to 180°C.

In a large bowl, whisk the eggs and milk together until combined. Season with salt and pepper, then add the remaining ingredients. Stir to mix.

Pour the mixture into greased muffin trays and cook for 15 minutes, or until frittatas are cooked through.

Serves 2

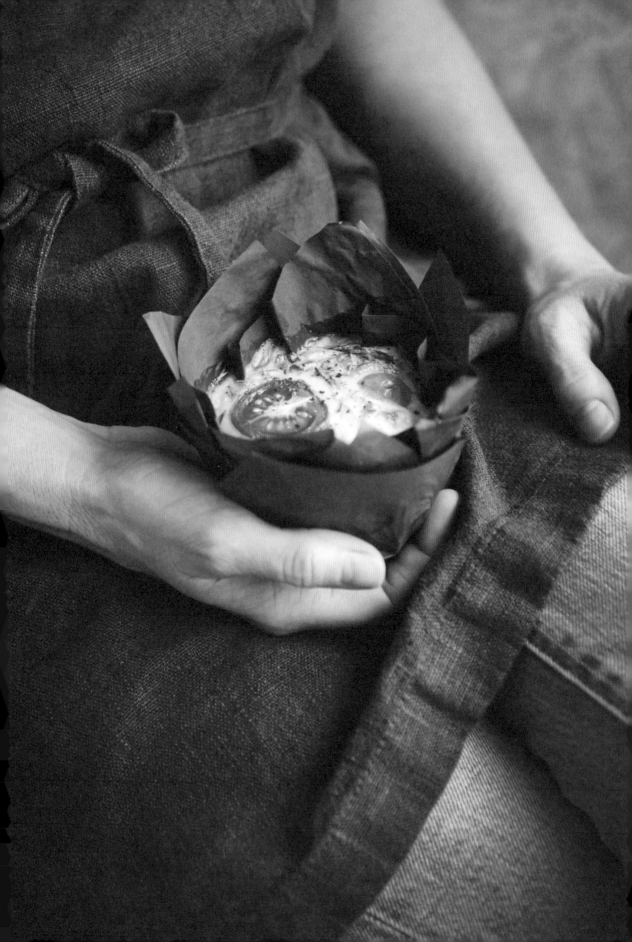

Quinoa Porridge

Sometimes in winter I have this every morning for brekky! I like to experiment with different toppings. For a treat, try adding a dollop of yoghurt on top with tahini drizzled over. Delish!

Ingredients

½ cup quinoa flakes

1 cup almond milk

1 tablespoon honey

½ teaspoon cinnamon

1 apple, grated

½ vanilla pod, seeds scraped out

sheep's milk yoghurt, for serving

strawberries, for serving

almonds, for serving

Place the quinoa, almond milk, honey and cinnamon in a saucepan over medium heat. Bring to the boil then reduce the heat, cover with a lid and simmer.

Once the quinoa is one-third of the way through cooking (check packet instructions), stir in the grated apple and vanilla seeds.

Once everything is cooked, place in a bowl. Garnish with a dollop of yoghurt and chopped strawberries and almonds. Sprinkle with cinnamon and drizzle with extra honey if you desire.

Serves 1

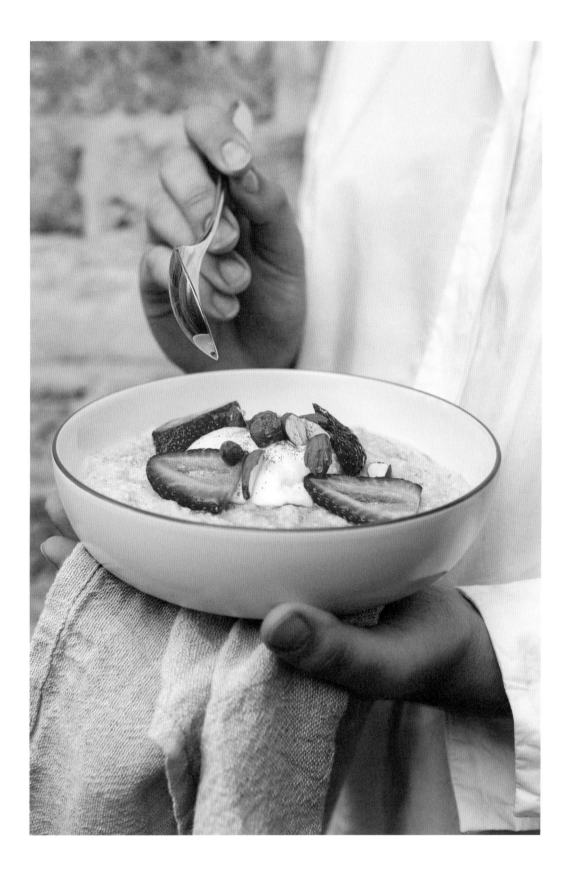

Omelette

A favourite at my place. Nutritious and a great way to fuel your body for a big day!

Ingredients

3 medium eggs

dash of milk (goat's, cow or sheep)

1 tablespoon olive oil

¼ long red chilli, deseeded

2 spring onions

¼ capsicum, deseeded and sliced

½ carrot, grated

½ zucchini, grated

butter, for cooking

handful baby spinach leaves

1 tablespoon goat's feta

salt and pepper

In a bowl, whisk the eggs and a dash of milk until combined.

Heat the olive oil in a frying pan over medium heat, add the chilli and spring onions, and stir until the spring onions are semi-cooked. Add the capsicum and cook for about 1 minute. Add the grated carrot and zucchini and sauté until soft. Once cooked, remove from the pan and place in a bowl.

Coat the frying pan with a bit of butter, ensuring the sides are also greased. Add the whisked egg. Place a lid over the frying pan and wait until the omelette is mostly cooked through. I always leave it a little bit undercooked on the top as it will continue to set when it's taken out of the pan.

Slide the omelette onto a plate. Place the vegetable mixture over half of the omelette, sprinkle with spinach, goat's feta, salt and pepper. Fold the rest of the omelette over the vegetable mixture and wham bam, thank you, ma'am you have yourself a fulfilling, nutritious breakfast that will keep you energised throughout the day.

Serves 1

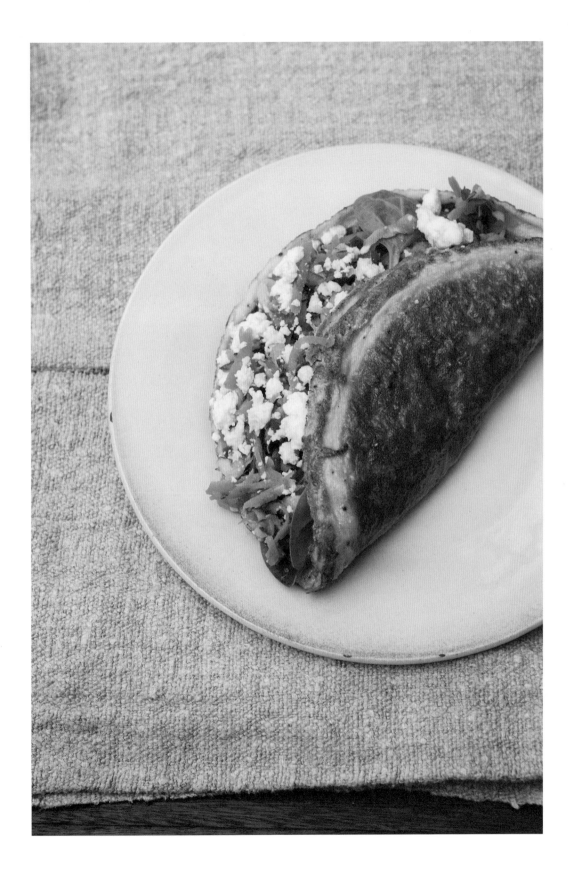

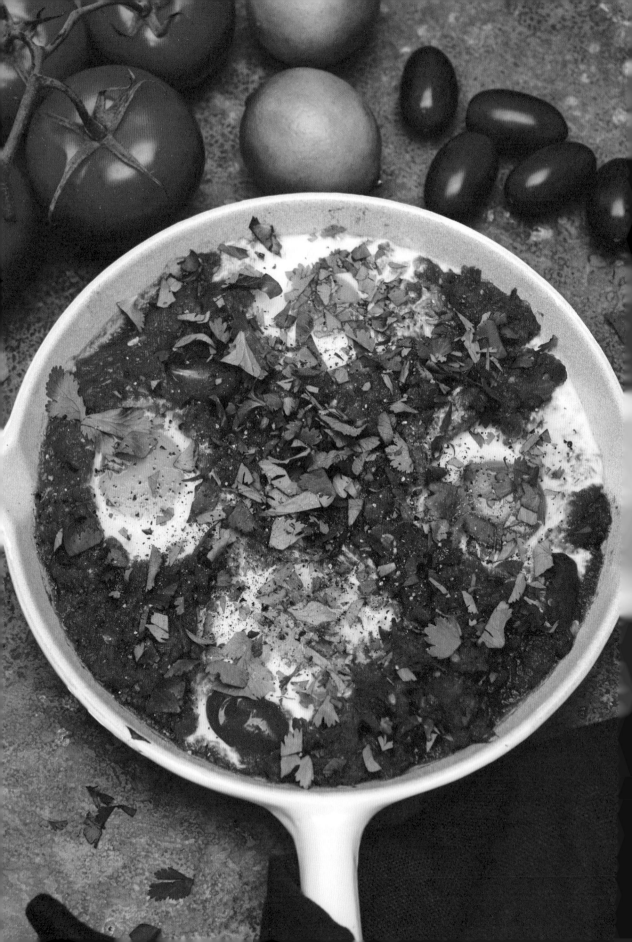

Baked Eggs in
Spicy Sauce

The perfect Sunday brekky.

Ingredients

6 tomatoes

2 small onions, peeled

6 cloves garlic, peeled

2 fresh red chillies

1 teaspoon ground cumin

2 teaspoons pink sea salt

4 medium eggs

juice of 1 lime

½ small bunch fresh coriander
leaves, chopped

Preheat the oven to 180°C.

Place the tomatoes, onion, garlic, red chilli (remove seeds if you prefer less heat), cumin and salt in a blender and blitz until smooth (but still a little chunky). You might like to add ½ cup water if it seems to be sticking – just to loosen it up a little.

Transfer the blended mix to a small saucepan and place over medium heat. Bring to a gentle simmer and reduce the sauce until it is nice and thick and fragrant, roughly 20 minutes. Pour this into a small, shallow baking dish (about 10cm round).

Crack the 4 eggs into the top of the dish so that they are nestled gently in the sauce, cover and place the dish in the oven. Cook for approximately 15–20 minutes or until eggs are set to your liking (I like the yolks to be oozy but the whites cooked all the way through).

Drizzle the cooked eggs with the lime juice and scatter with chopped coriander leaves to serve.

Serves 2

Sweet Potato Fritters

These are my healthy hash browns!

Ingredients

1 large sweet potato

4 large eggs

1 teaspoon pink sea salt

1 red long chilli, finely diced,
to taste

1 clove garlic, peeled and finely
diced, to taste

2 tablespoons olive oil

Peel and grate the sweet potato (it should make roughly 3 cups of grated goodness). Squeeze the grated sweet potato over the sink to remove all the excess moisture; use muslin or cheesecloth if you have it, or a clean stocking.

In a large bowl, whisk the eggs, add the sweet potato and sea salt, and chilli and garlic if using. Mix well to combine.

Heat the olive oil in a frying pan over medium heat – you'll know the pan is hot enough if there is a satisfying sizzle when the mix hits the oil. Add large dollops of the sweet potato mix to the pan – they should be about 6–7cm wide and about ½–1cm thick. Make sure the fritters aren't too thick or they won't cook all the way through. Cook for 2–3 minutes on each side until nicely caramelised. Remove the fritters to a plate lined with paper towel to drain any excess oil.

Serve with the Guacamole – you can find that recipe on the next page.

Makes about 10 fritters

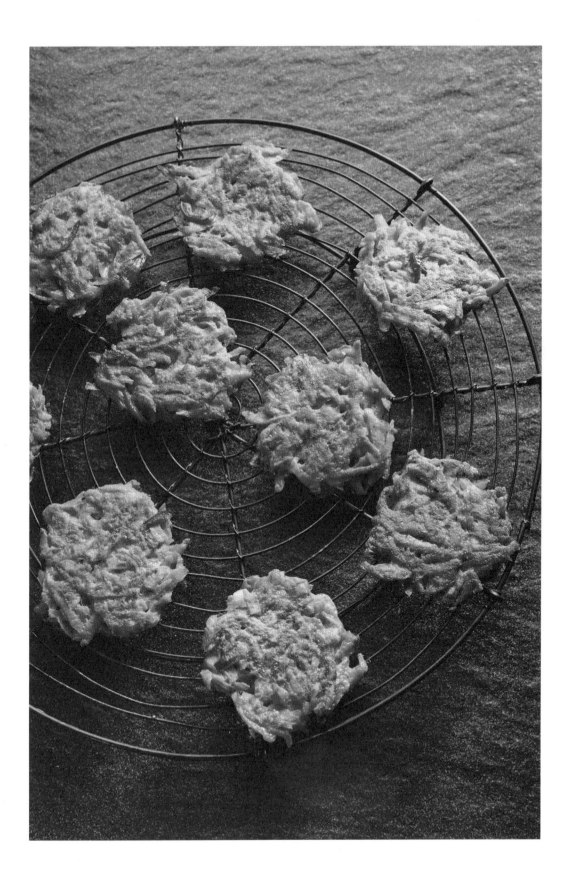

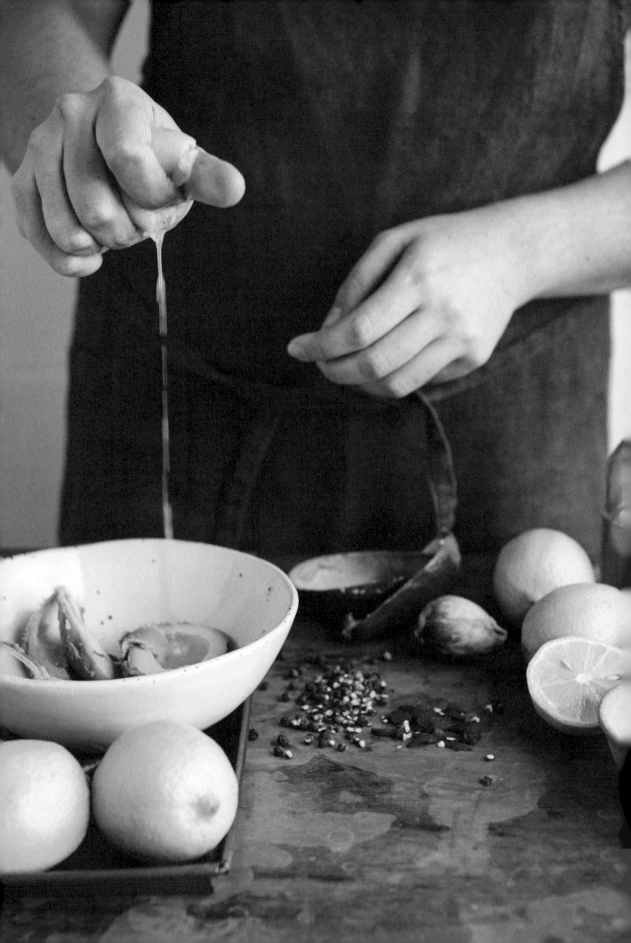

Guacamole

Guac makes everything taste better! I always have some made up in my fridge. I put it on my eggs in the morning, add it to a salad or simply dip some veg sticks in it for an easy snack.

Ingredients

2 medium avocados

juice of ½ lemon

dash of olive oil

1 fresh chilli, finely sliced

pinch of pink sea salt

Cut the avocados in half. Remove the pit and scoop out the flesh into a bowl. Mash with a fork until it becomes chunky.

Add the lemon juice and stir to make the consistency smooth. Add the smallest dash of olive oil, chilli (remove the seeds if you prefer less heat) and sea salt, and mix through.

Holy guacamole, you can thank me later.

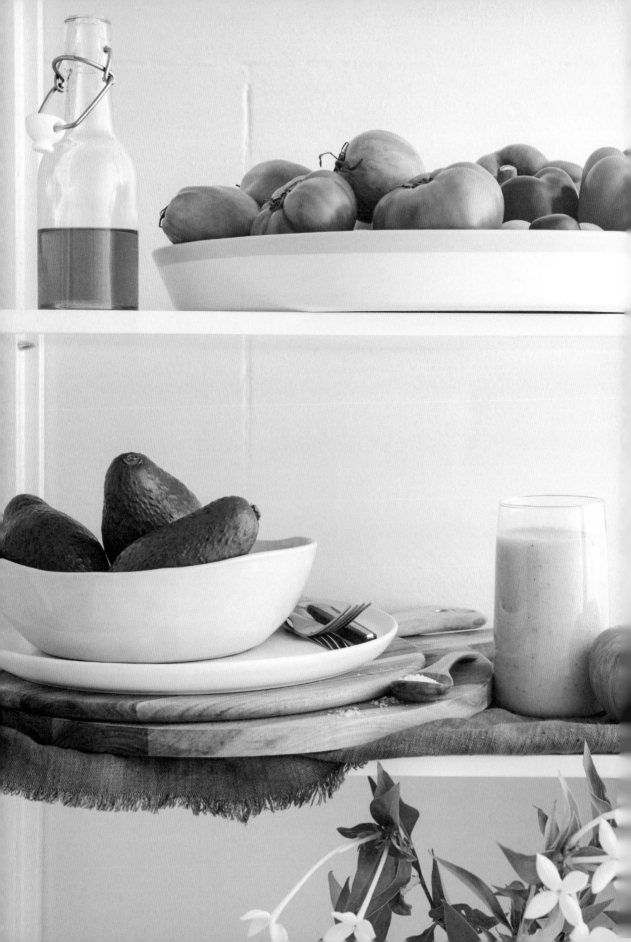

Lunch

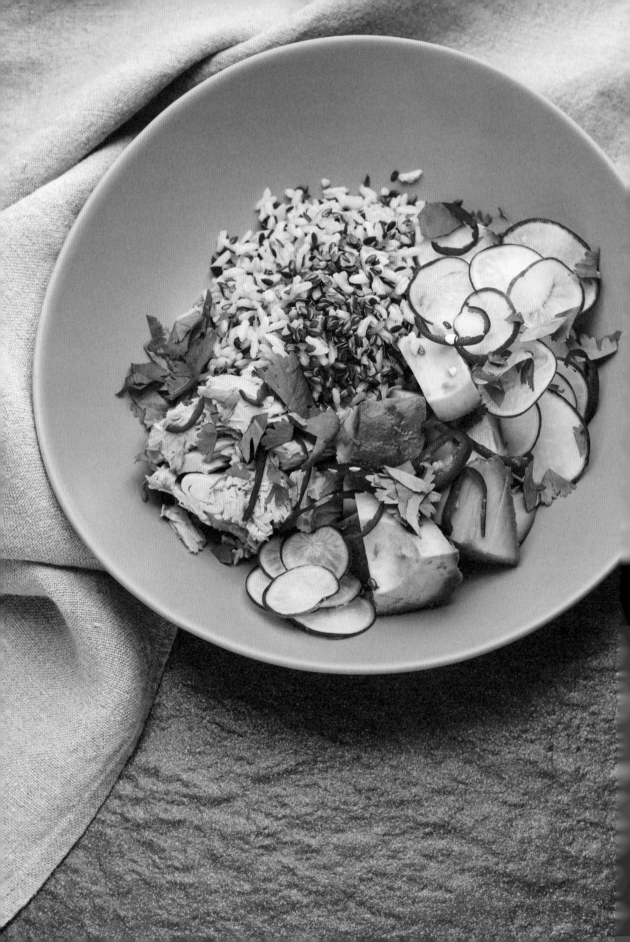

Avocado, Tuna and
Brown Rice Bowl

Quick 'n' easy! This lunch has everything I need in it –
the brown rice provides me with good carbohydrates,
the tuna is my protein and the avo covers my good fats
and omegas!

Ingredients

½ cup brown rice

¼ cup flaxseeds

95g tin of tuna in springwater

1 medium avocado

1 small bunch radishes

½ bunch fresh coriander leaves,
   roughly chopped

½ small fresh red chilli, finely
   chopped

juice of 1 lime

1 tablespoon olive oil

salt and pepper

Place the brown rice in a small saucepan with
2–2½ cups of water. Bring to a gentle simmer
over a low to medium heat and cover with a lid.
Leave gently bubbling for about 35 minutes. By
this time all the water should be absorbed and
the rice should be perfectly *al dente*. Check it
occasionally to make sure it isn't boiling too
fast and absorbing the water too quickly.

Mix the cooked brown rice with the flaxseeds.
Drain the tuna, add to the brown rice mixture
and place in a small serving bowl.

Chop the avocado flesh into roughly 1½cm
cubes. Slice the radishes thinly into circles.
Place the avocado and radish in a bowl with the
coriander, chilli, lime juice and olive oil, and
mix these all together.

Top the brown rice mix with the avocado
salad and season with salt and pepper to taste.

Serves 1

TIP: I LEAVE THE SEEDS IN THE CHILLI, BUT TAKE
THEM OUT IF THEY'RE TOO SPICY FOR YOU.

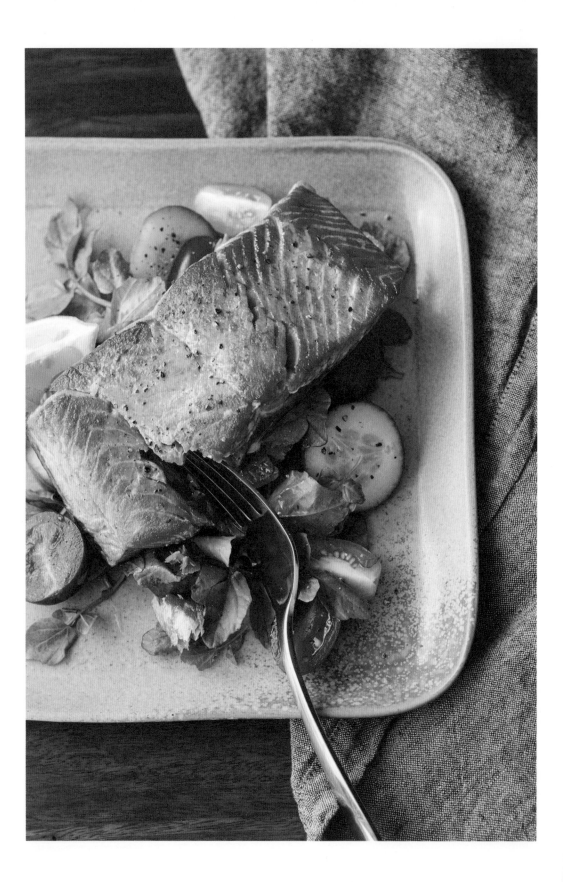

Seared Salmon with
Watercress Salad

Simply delicious! Sometimes less is more. I love salmon prepared like this.

Ingredients

1 fresh salmon fillet, approx. 200g

pinch of pink sea salt

1–2 tablespoons olive oil

½ bunch fresh watercress

½ punnet cherry tomatoes

1 medium Lebanese cucumber

juice of ½ lemon

extra olive oil, for dressing

salt and pepper

Preheat the oven to 180°C.

Season the salmon fillet with a pinch of salt. Place a frying pan over medium heat and add the olive oil. When the pan is hot, place the salmon flesh side down in the pan – if it's hot enough it should make a satisfying sizzling sound. Cook for about 2 minutes or until nicely caramelised on that side. Flip and cook the skin side of the fillet for about 30 seconds. Transfer the fillet to a baking tray and place in the oven for 3–4 minutes to cook through. Remove from the oven and place the fillet on paper towel to rest.

Meanwhile, wash the watercress under running water then shake the excess moisture out over the sink. Roughly chop the watercress. Halve the cherry tomatoes and dice the cucumber into satisfying chunks. Toss the watercress, tomatoes and cucumber in a bowl with the lemon juice and a splash of olive oil.

To serve, place the salmon on a bed of salad and season with salt and pepper to taste.

Serves 1

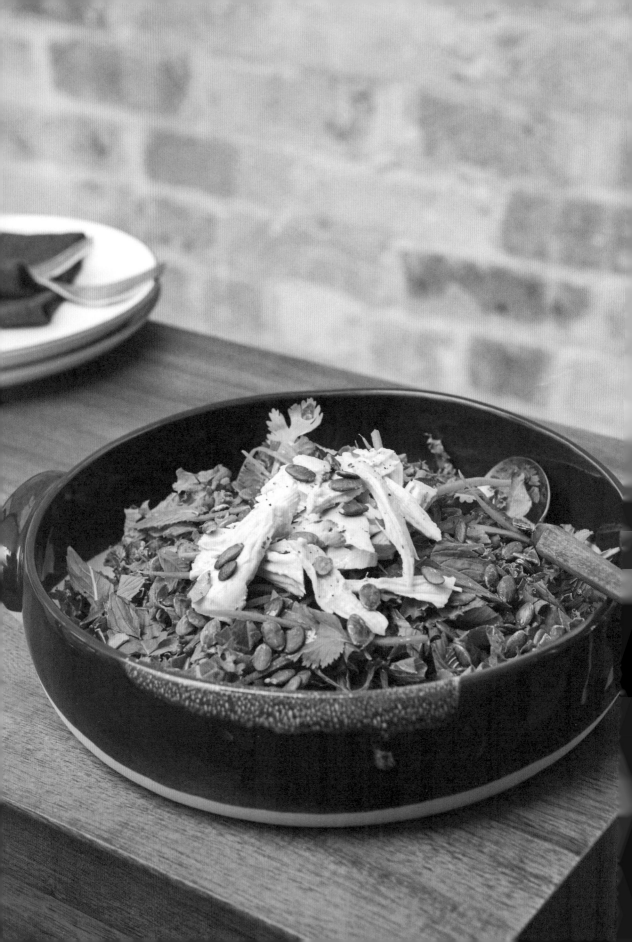

Leftover Poached Chicken Salad

I'm the queen of leftovers! It saves loads of time and makes meal prep so quick. I love the texture and crunch of this salad.

Ingredients

leftover turmeric poached chicken (see recipe page 204)

small handful kale

½ bunch fresh mint leaves

½ bunch fresh coriander leaves

1 small carrot

1 fresh red chilli

juice of 1 lime

dash of olive oil

2 tablespoons toasted pumpkin seeds

salt and pepper

Thinly slice or shred the leftover turmeric poached chicken (or cook according to recipe on page 204).

Wash and roughly chop the kale, mint and coriander. Peel and thinly slice or grate the carrot, and thinly slice the red chilli (remove seeds if you don't like it too hot). Combine the salad ingredients in a bowl or on a plate, then dress with the lime juice and olive oil.

To serve, place the poached chicken on a bed of salad, then scatter with toasted pumpkin seeds. Season with salt and pepper to taste.

Serves 1

Chilli Oil Tuna Salad

Another easy salad I can make on set. I just pack tuna, avo and a bag of spinach leaves in my bag and make it all up in a matter of minutes!

Ingredients

95g tin of tuna in springwater

½ medium avocado

1 Lebanese cucumber

1 small red onion (optional)

1 cup baby spinach leaves

1 tablespoon apple cider vinegar

2 tablespoons chilli oil

salt and pepper

Drain the tuna and place in a serving bowl. Roughly chop the avocado and cucumber into chunky cubes. Peel and finely chop the red onion if using. Add to the bowl with the tuna and baby spinach leaves.

Dress the salad with the vinegar and chilli oil. Season with salt and pepper to taste.

Serves 1

TIP: SOMETIMES IF I'M FEELING QUITE HUNGRY, I'LL ADD ½ CUP COOKED BROWN RICE AND SOME NUTS OR SEEDS TO THIS SALAD. PLAY AROUND WITH IT, IT'S QUITE DELICIOUS.

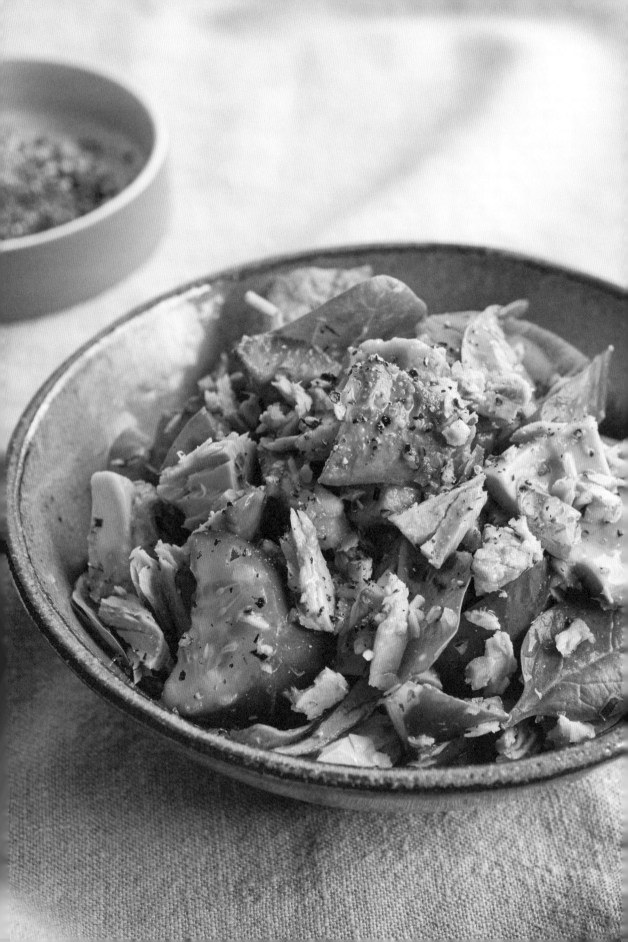

Boiled Eggs with
Blanched Greens and Nuts

I always feel so good after having this for lunch! It makes me feel satisfied but without that heavy, full feeling.

Ingredients

2 large eggs

1 small bunch bok choy or choy sum

⅓ cup toasted unsalted almonds, roughly chopped

⅓ cup toasted unsalted cashews, roughly chopped

1 tablespoon olive oil

salt and pepper

Bring a saucepan of water to the boil. Add the eggs and boil for 1 minute. Turn off the heat and leave the eggs in the hot water for 10 minutes. Remove the eggs and place them in a small bowl of cold water. When the shells have cooled, peel the eggs and put them aside.

Bring a saucepan of water to the boil again. Place the greens in the boiling water and briskly simmer, uncovered. Using a slotted spoon, remove the greens from the water as soon as they have softened – only a couple of minutes at most; any longer and they'll turn to mush. Rinse them in a bowl of cold water to stop the cooking process. Drain the leaves and place them in a serving bowl.

Roughly chop the eggs then place in the bowl with the blanched greens. Add the toasted nuts, dress with olive oil, and toss to combine. Season with salt and pepper to taste.

Serves 1

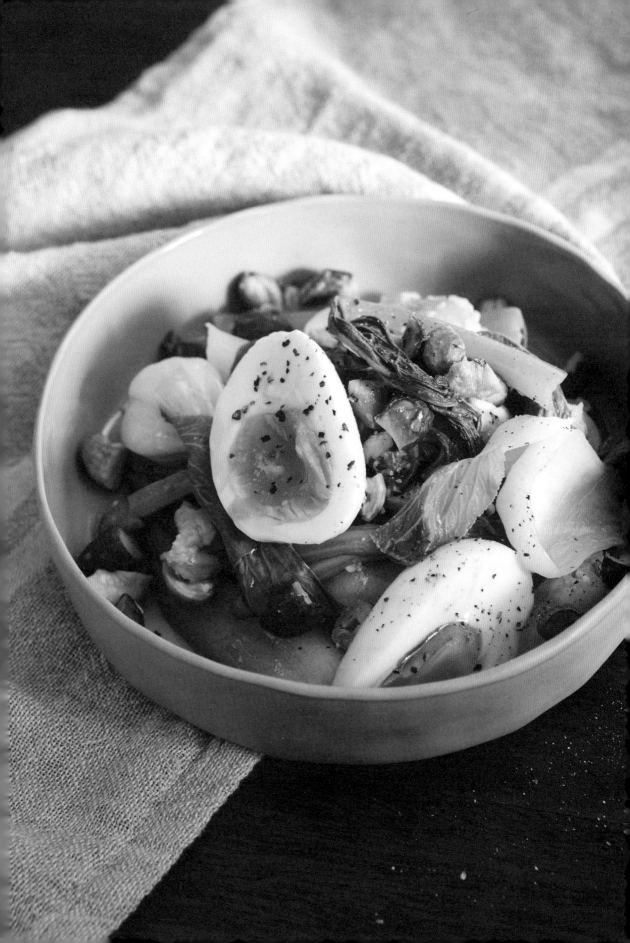

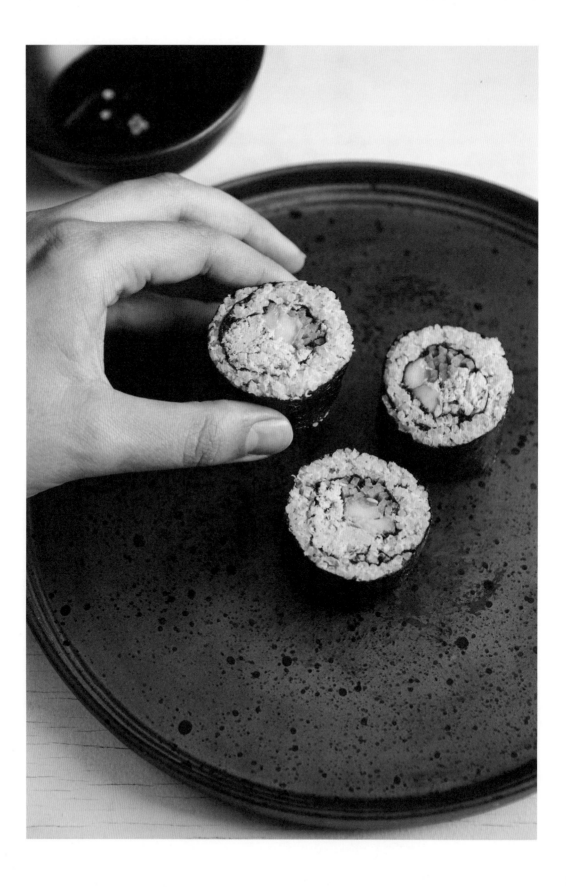

Quinoa & Tahini Sushi

Ingredients

1½ cups quinoa

1 tablespoon tahini

1 tablespoon rice wine vinegar

1 tablespoon toasted sesame
seeds

2 × 95g tins of tuna in
springwater

1 small to medium avocado,
finely sliced

2 Lebanese cucumbers, cut into
thin strips

1 carrot, cut into thin strips

1 pack nori sheets

chilli oil, for serving (optional)

hummus, for serving (optional)

Rinse the quinoa thoroughly, cook according
to packet instructions and then allow to cool.
Mix the cooled quinoa with the tahini, rice wine
vinegar and sesame seeds.

Drain the tuna and roughly mash. Place the
avocado, cucumber and carrot into bowls for
easy access as you roll your sushi. You may
also like to have a small bowl of water handy to
rinse your fingers.

If you have a sushi mat, place one sheet
of nori on the mat – or place the nori sheet
directly on a chopping board. Spread some of
the quinoa mixture over the nori sheet, press
down quite firmly so it's slightly compacted.
Leave a small border along the edge furthest
away from you. How thick you make the quinoa
is up to you, but a thinner layer of 2–3mm will
be easier to roll.

Place a few slices of avocado, cucumber
and carrot along the middle of the sheet
lengthways, and then add a line of mashed
tuna. Roll up the nori sheet away from you,
trying to keep the fillings tightly within the
wrapper. Brush a little water along the edge to
help the sheet stick together.

Repeat to make as many rolls as you like.
You can slice the rolls if desired – using a
clean knife, cut the roll in half or into bite-
sized pieces. I like to dip these in chilli oil or
hummus – or simply have them on their own.

Serves 2

Seared Tuna with
Zucchini Noodles

Ingredients

1 fresh tuna fillet, approx. 200g

pinch of pink sea salt

1–2 tablespoons olive oil

1 large zucchini

3 squash

1cm piece fresh ginger, peeled
  and finely grated

1 fresh red chilli

juice of 1 lemon

extra olive oil, for dressing

salt and pepper

Preheat the oven to 180°C.

Season the tuna fillet with a pinch of salt. Place a frying pan over medium heat and add the olive oil. When the pan is hot, place the fillet in the pan – it should make a satisfying sizzling sound. Cook for about 2 minutes or until nicely caramelised on that side. Flip and cook on the other side for about 30 seconds. Transfer the fillet to a baking tray and place in the oven for 3–4 minutes to cook through. Remove from the oven and place the fillet on paper towel to rest.

Meanwhile, cut the ends off the zucchini and finely shave into long slices with a vegetable peeler, or run it through a spiralizer. Cut the squash into halves or quarters. Bring a small saucepan of water to the boil, add the zucchini strips and squash, and cook for 3–4 minutes or until the veggies are as soft as you like them. Immediately drain and rinse with cold water to stop the cooking process, then drain well.

Finely slice the red chilli (remove the seeds if you don't want it too hot). In a bowl, toss the zucchini, squash, ginger and chilli with the lemon juice and a dash of olive oil. Serve the tuna fillet on a bed of zucchini noodles and season with salt and pepper to taste.

Serves 1

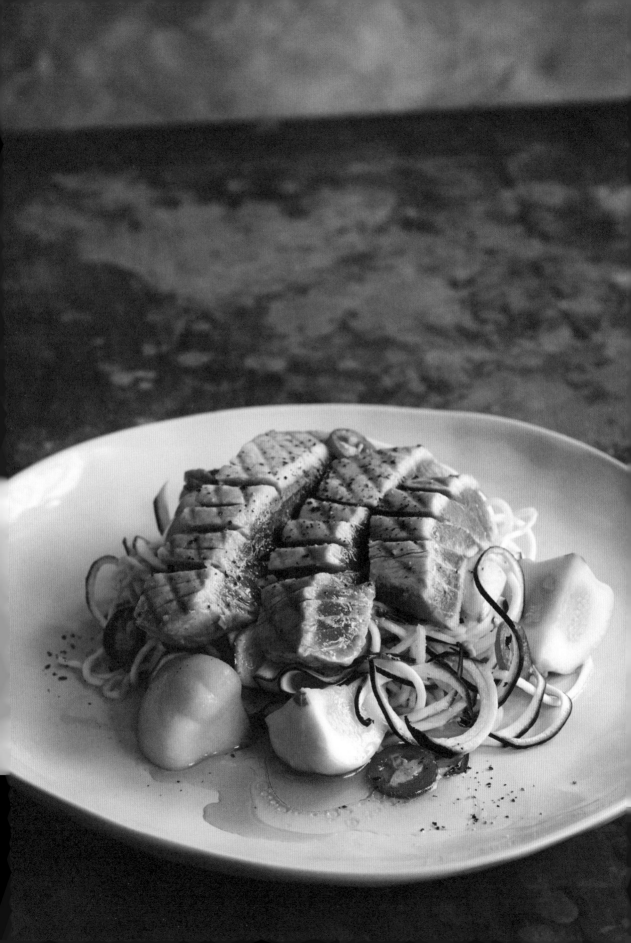

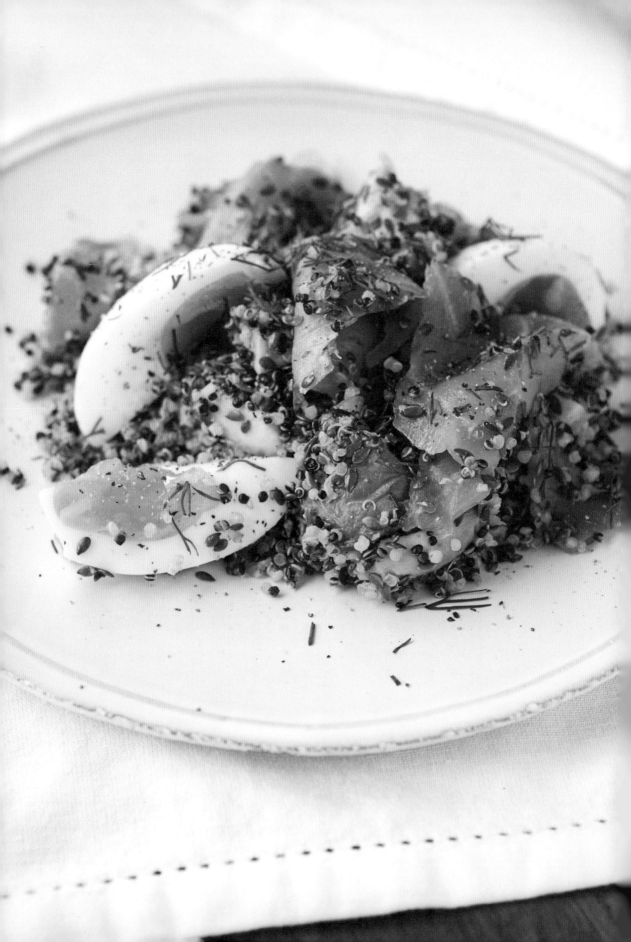

Smoked Salmon with
Egg, Avocado and Quinoa

I love brekky so much I found out how to get away with having it for lunch.

Ingredients

½ cup quinoa

¼ cup flaxseeds

1 tablespoon apple cider vinegar

2 medium eggs

200g smoked salmon

1 medium avocado

½ cup fresh dill, finely chopped

salt and pepper

Rinse the quinoa thoroughly and cook according to packet instructions. Allow the cooked quinoa to cool then mix with the flaxseeds and vinegar and set aside.

Meanwhile, bring a saucepan of water to the boil. Add the eggs and boil for 1 minute. Turn off the heat and leave the eggs in the hot water for 10 minutes. Remove the eggs and place in a small bowl of cold water. When the shells have cooled, peel the eggs and set aside.

Roughly chop the smoked salmon, avocado and boiled eggs. Toss with the quinoa mixture and scatter with the fresh dill. Season with salt and pepper to taste.

Serves 2

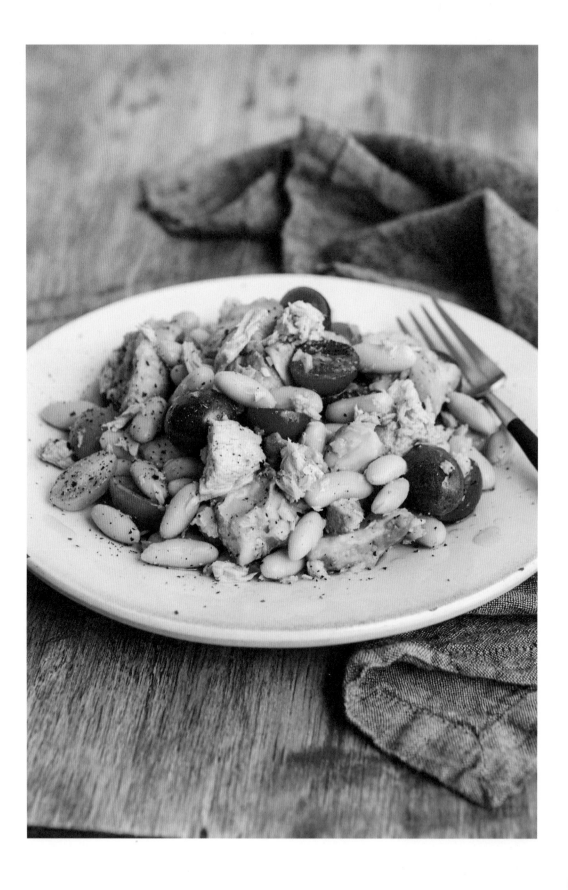

Bean & Tuna Salad

Simple and full of flavour!

Ingredients

95g tin of tuna in springwater

400g tin of cannellini beans

½ medium avocado

½ punnet cherry tomatoes

juice of ½ lemon

1cm piece fresh ginger, peeled
and finely grated

1 tablespoon olive oil

salt and pepper

Drain the tuna and cannellini beans, place in a bowl and toss together. Roughly chop the avocado, halve the tomatoes and toss through the tuna and bean mix.

In a small bowl, mix the lemon juice, grated ginger and olive oil. Season the dressing with salt and pepper to taste. Toss the salad with the dressing and serve.

Serves 1

Roasted Sweet Potato and
Kale Salad

Health and happiness all in one bowl!

Ingredients

1 large sweet potato

3 cloves garlic

2 or 3 stalks fresh rosemary

1 teaspoon pink sea salt

2 tablespoons olive oil

1 small bunch kale

1 tablespoon apple cider vinegar

extra olive oil, for dressing

2 tablespoons toasted pumpkin
seeds

Preheat the oven to 180°C.

Peel and chop the sweet potato into 1cm dice. Peel and finely grate or chop the garlic. Finely chop the leaves of the rosemary stalks. In a bowl, toss together the sweet potato, garlic, rosemary, sea salt and 2 tablespoons olive oil.

Scatter the dressed sweet potato over the base of a large roasting pan so that the pieces are not crowded. Bake for about 35–40 minutes or until the sweet potato is nicely roasted and soft but crisp on the outside.

Roughly chop the kale and dress with the vinegar and extra olive oil. Serve the sweet potato on a bed of kale and scatter with the toasted pumpkin seeds.

Serves 1–2

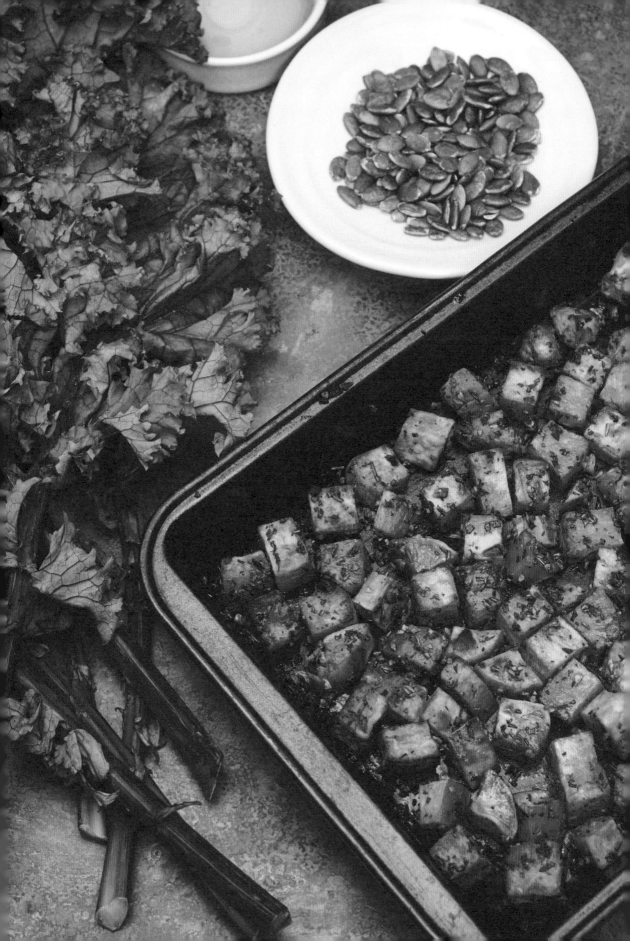

Roasted Brussels Sprout Salad

Didn't like Brussels sprouts as a kid? This salad will change your mind.

Ingredients

10–12 medium Brussels sprouts, halved

3 cloves garlic

2 tablespoons olive oil

½ bunch kale

juice of 1 lemon

extra olive oil, for dressing

1 cup toasted walnuts, roughly chopped

salt and pepper

Preheat the oven to 180°C.

Peel and finely grate or chop the garlic cloves. In a small bowl, toss together the sprouts, garlic and 2 tablespoons olive oil.

Scatter the sprouts over the base of a roasting tin. Bake for 10–15 minutes or until the sprouts are nicely browned on top.

Roughly chop the kale and dress in the lemon juice and a dash of olive oil. Mix the roasted sprouts with the kale and serve in a bowl scattered with the chopped walnuts. Season with salt and pepper to taste.

Serves 2

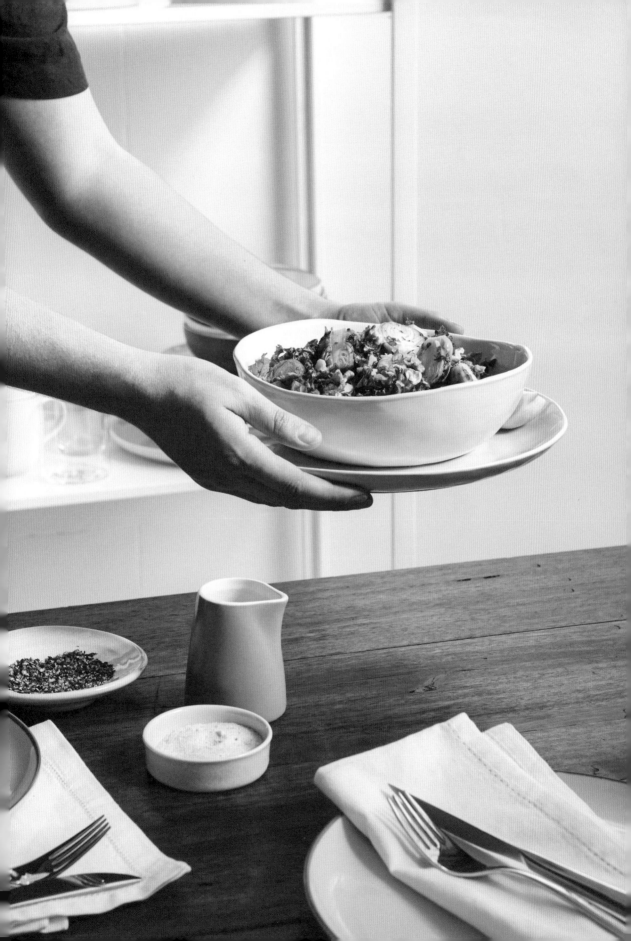

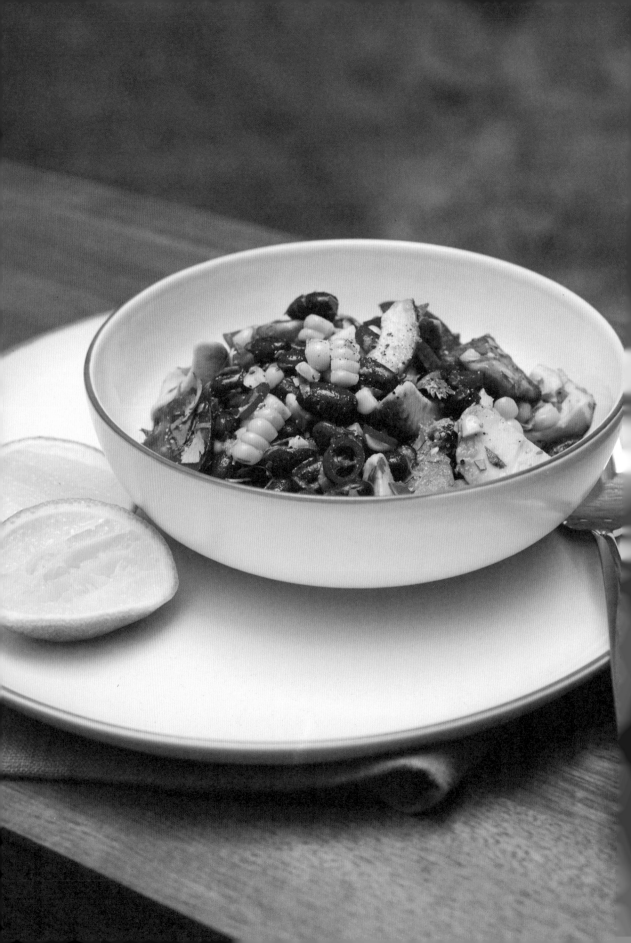

Mexican Avocado Salad

I fell in love with Mexican flavours after a holiday to Cabo years ago. Fresh and tasty, this takes me straight back to the long summer days I spent on the beach.

Ingredients

1 cob fresh corn, husk removed

125g tin red kidney beans

1 medium avocado

1 medium tomato

1 small bunch fresh coriander

1 small fresh red chilli

zest and juice of 1 lime

½ teaspoon ground cumin

salt and pepper

Bring a small saucepan of water to the boil and add the corn cob. Turn off the heat and let the corn cook in the hot water for 10 minutes. Drain the corn and allow to cool slightly. Using a sharp knife, cut the corn kernels from the cob and set aside.

Drain the red kidney beans. Roughly chop the avocado and tomato. Finely chop the coriander (including the stalks). Mix the corn, beans, avocado, tomato and coriander together in a serving bowl.

Finely chop the chilli (remove seeds if you don't like it too hot), place in a small bowl with the lime zest, lime juice and cumin, and mix well. Add to the salad and combine all ingredients. Season with salt and pepper to taste.

Serves 1

TIP: IF YOU CAN LEAVE THIS LOVELY SALAD IN THE FRIDGE OVERNIGHT, IT ONLY GETS BETTER.

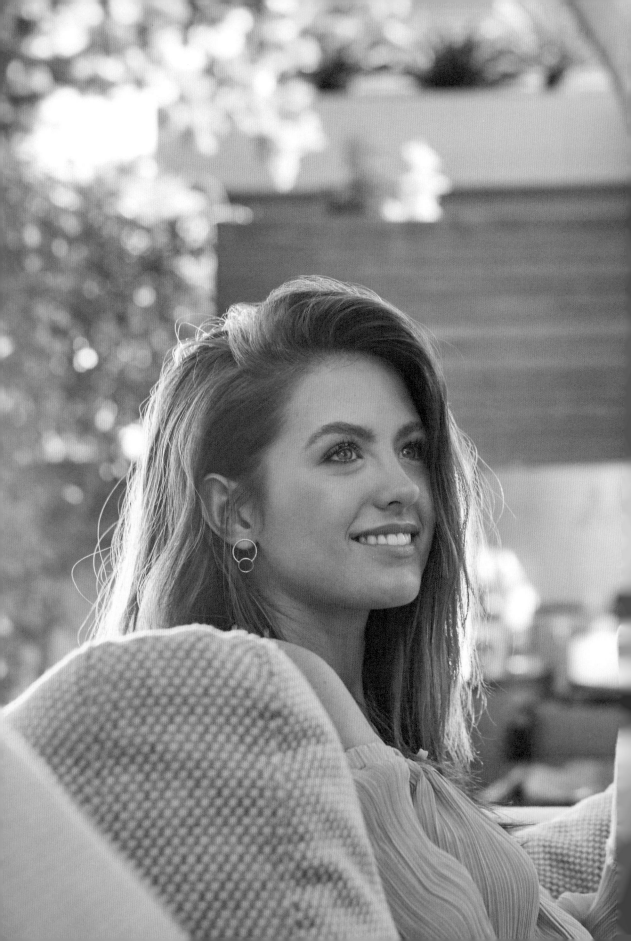

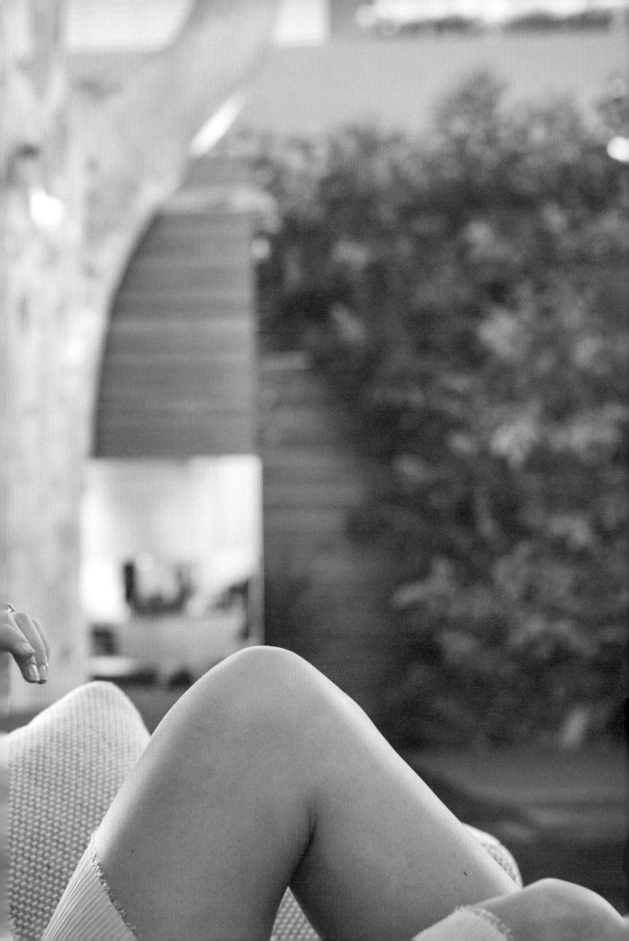

Dinner

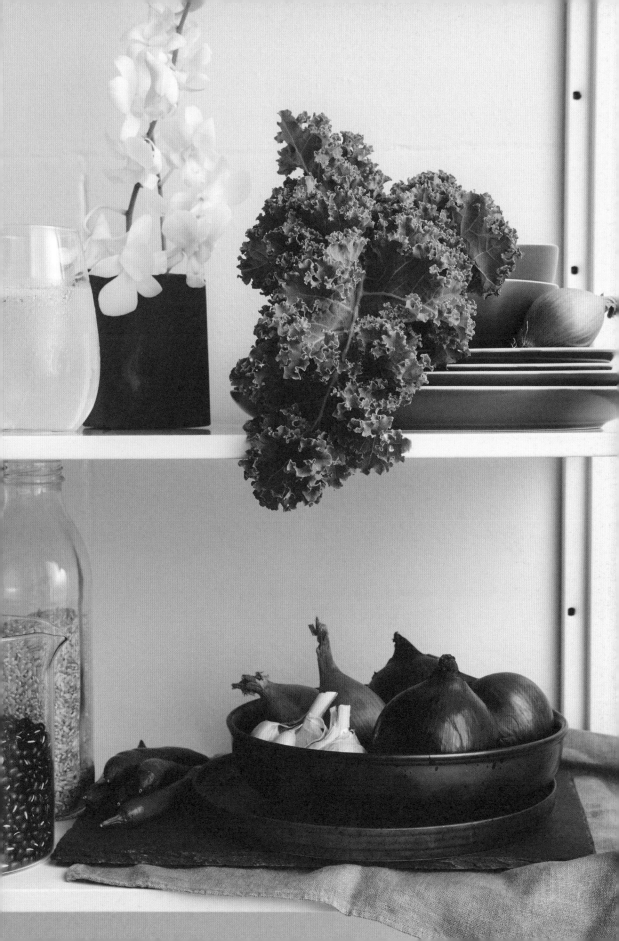

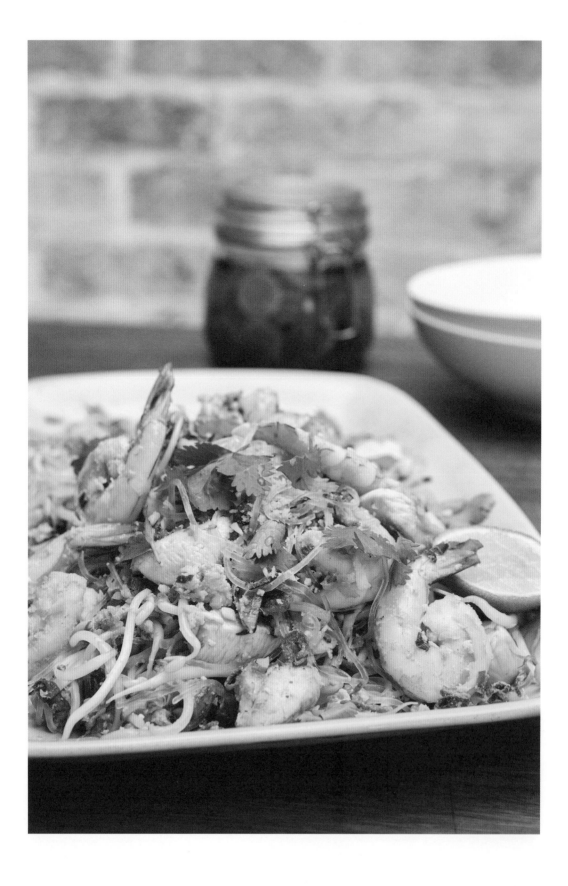

Pad Thai with *Kelp Noodles*

When I was in Thailand with *Getaway* we filmed a segment for the show at a cooking school. I learnt how to make many of my favourite Thai dishes and this pad Thai is one of them. I've altered the recipe a little bit and use kelp noodles to suit my way of eating.

Ingredients

1 tablespoon coconut oil

100g chicken breast fillet or tofu, cut into cubes

3 spring onions, finely chopped

2 tablespoons pickled radish, chopped

10 uncooked prawns, peeled

2 medium eggs, beaten

2 tablespoons dried shrimp

4 teaspoons honey

1–2 teaspoons lime juice (to taste, try 1 teaspoon and add by halves if you want more)

1 tablespoon fish sauce

2–3 tablespoons roasted peanuts, finely ground

1 long red chilli, finely chopped (if you love it spicy, add two)

1 cup bean sprouts

454g packet kelp noodles

fresh coriander leaves, to garnish

Heat the coconut oil in a wok or large frying pan over high heat. Add the chicken or tofu and stir-fry until cooked. Remove and place on paper towel to drain.

To the same wok, add the spring onions, pickled radish and prawns, and stir-fry until prawns turn pink and are cooked.

Add the eggs and cook for a few seconds. Then add the dried shrimp and the chicken or tofu, and cook for about 45 seconds. Add the honey, lime juice, fish sauce, roasted peanuts and chilli, and stir-fry for a good minute. Add the bean sprouts and kelp noodles and mix to combine. Cook until the kelp noodles are a little bit soft. Garnish with fresh coriander before serving.

Serves 2

TIP: MOST TRADITIONAL THAI RECIPES USE SUGAR, BUT I PREFER HONEY FOR A DELICIOUS FLAVOUR.

Chicken & Vegetable Curry

Curry is my go-to winter meal. I've visited India twice and can't wait to go back again purely for the food. Until then, this curry will have to do.

Ingredients

1 carrot

1 zucchini

¼ head broccoli

½ sweet potato, peeled

2 chicken breast fillets

1–2 tablespoons olive oil

1 teaspoon finely diced fresh chilli

½ capsicum, deseeded and finely diced

1 white onion, peeled and finely diced

4 teaspoons green curry paste

handful green beans, halved

270ml can coconut cream

¾ cup coconut milk

pinch of pink sea salt

pepper

cooked brown or white rice or quinoa, for serving

Chop the carrot, zucchini, broccoli and sweet potato into chunks. It doesn't have to look pretty, I like big chunks of veggies in my curry. Cut the chicken breast into 3–5cm pieces.

In a large frying pan or pot, heat the olive oil over medium heat. Add the chilli, capsicum and onion. When the onion becomes clear, add the chicken. Sear the chicken then add the curry paste. Mix until the chicken is coated in the curry paste. Add all of the vegetables and stir through. Add the coconut cream and coconut milk, stir to mix, and reduce the heat so the sauce is just simmering. Place the lid on the pan or pot and leave to cook through for about 30 minutes or until vegetables are soft. Season with salt and pepper.

Serve with cooked brown or white rice or quinoa.

Serves 2

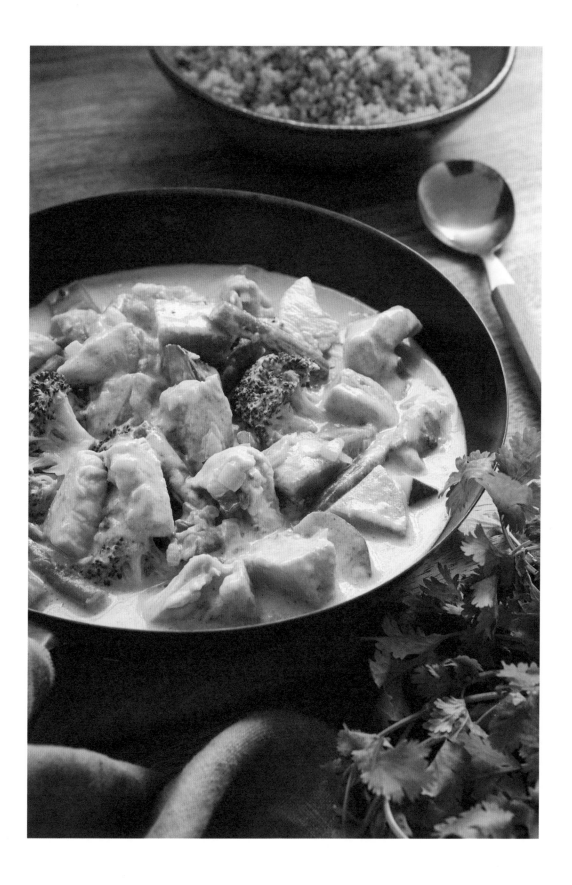

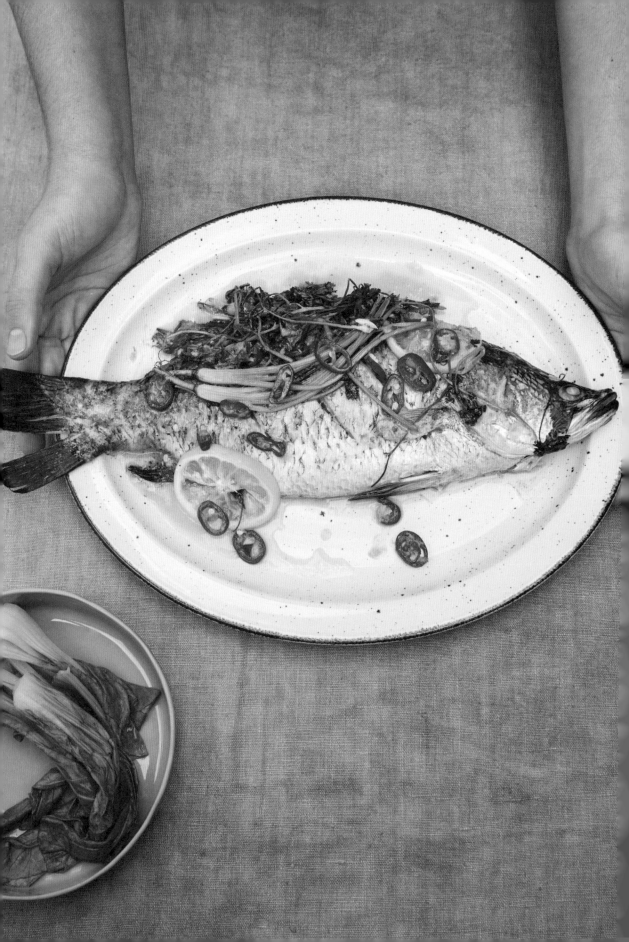

Whole Baked Barramundi

A great dish to share with your family or friends.

Ingredients

120g butter

1 fresh chilli, sliced

1 lemon, zested

1 whole barramundi, descaled

pinch of pink sea salt

1 bunch fresh coriander

cracked black pepper

steamed green veggies, for
  serving

Preheat the oven to 180°C.

Melt the butter in a small saucepan over low heat. Add the chilli and the zest of half the lemon and cook until you can smell their fragrance. Remove the pan from the heat and set aside.

Place the whole barramundi on a generous amount of foil in a baking tray. Rub the skin with a little pink sea salt. Pour the butter mixture over the fish. Slice the lemon into generous pieces and place all around fish. Cover with the bunch of coriander and season with cracked pepper. Wrap the fish up in the foil and bake in the oven for 30–40 minutes, depending on the size of the fish.

Serve with steamed green veggies.

Serves 2

Roasted Leg of Lamb

I often cook this when I have friends over for dinner. With a glass of red wine and a deck of cards, you're in for a good night.

Ingredients

2kg leg of lamb

2 tablespoons olive oil

salt and pepper

1 teaspoon ground cumin

1 teaspoon cumin seeds

2 red onions, peeled and sliced

¼ cup red wine

tomatoes on vine, mixed sizes

5 cloves garlic, skin on

3 bay leaves

1 teaspoon grated fresh ginger

handful fresh coriander leaves, for garnish

sprinkle of goat's feta, for garnish

Preheat the oven to 230°C.

Take your lamb and massage it with 2 tablespoons olive oil – really give it some good ol' loving! Season with a generous amount of salt and pepper and the ground cumin and cumin seeds.

Cover the base of a roasting tray with sliced onions and place the lamb on top. Cook in the oven for 30 minutes. Reduce the oven temperature to 180°C, add the wine to the tray and cook for a further 30 minutes. Add the tomatoes, garlic, bay leaves and ginger and cook for a further 20–30 minutes.

Remove the lamb from the oven, cover with foil and rest for 20 minutes.

Place in a serving dish, garnish with fresh coriander and goat's feta and serve.

Serves 3–4

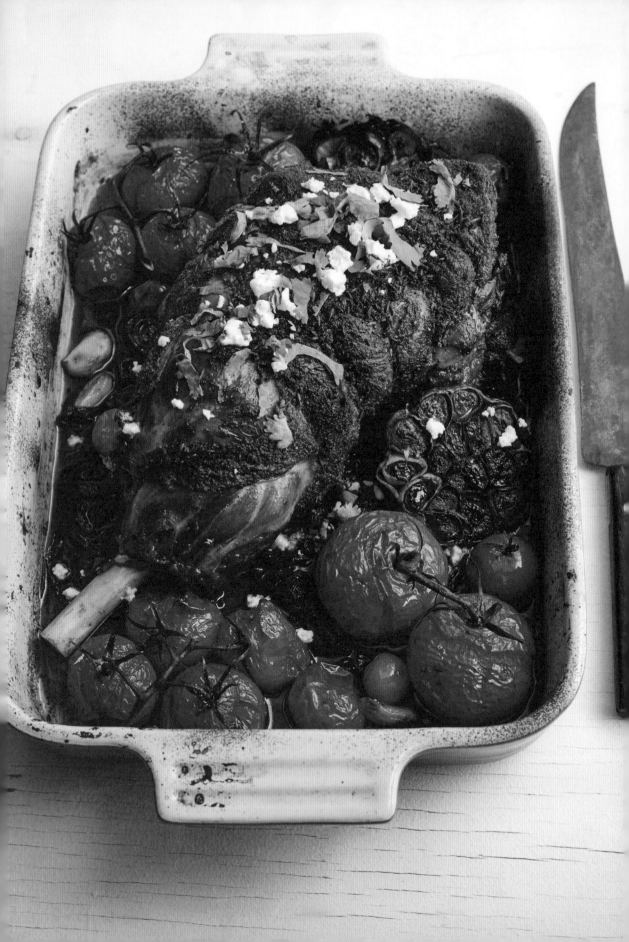

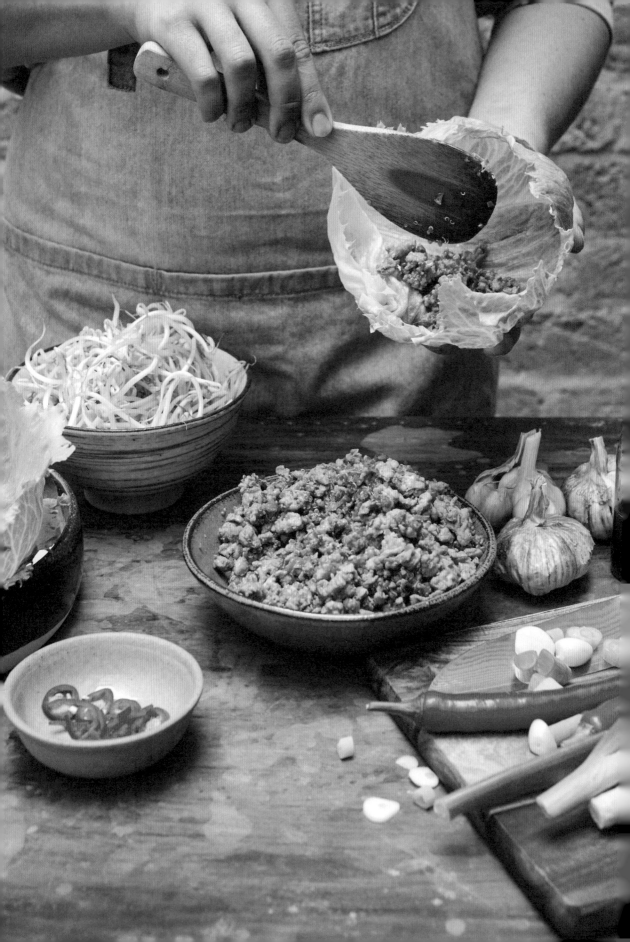

San Choy Bow

A favourite in my household for dinner! It never disappoints.

Ingredients

1 cup cooked quinoa

1 tablespoon coconut oil

2 cloves garlic, peeled and finely chopped

3 spring onions, sliced

1 long red chilli

1 stalk lemongrass, finely grated

1 packet chicken mince, approx. 500g

2 tablespoons tamari

2 dashes sesame oil

iceberg lettuce cups, for serving

handful bean sprouts, for serving

Cook the quinoa according to the packet instructions and set aside.

In a wok or frying pan over high heat, heat the coconut oil. Add the garlic and spring onions, stir and cook for about 45 seconds. Add the chilli and lemongrass, and cook until fragrant.

Add the chicken mince and stir until the chicken is about half cooked.

Stir in the cooked quinoa, tamari and 2 dashes of sesame oil, and cook until chicken is cooked through – no pink bits!

Serve in lettuce cups topped with bean sprouts.

Serves 3–4

Roasted Tofu

I love this recipe because it's so quick and easy and is great if you're time-poor. I don't eat lots of tofu as I try to minimise the amount of soy in my diet. I do love it as an alternative to meat, though, and I find it a great addition to salads and stir-fries, as long as I'm not eating it every day and balancing it with other sources of protein. I think too much of anything isn't good for you, and I wouldn't recommend replacing meats with just soy-based products – try to have a wide variety of non-meat options in your diet.

Ingredients

500g firm tofu

2 tablespoons tamari

1 tablespoon maple syrup

1 long red chilli, including seeds, finely sliced

1 tablespoon sesame seeds

2 cloves garlic, peeled and grated or finely diced

Preheat the oven to 180°C.

Chop the tofu into cubes and set aside.

Place the tamari, maple syrup, chilli, sesame seeds and garlic in a bowl. Whisk until combined.

Place the tofu in the tamari mix and toss to coat all over. You can either roast the tofu straightaway or leave it to marinate for between 30 minutes and 2 hours.

Spread the tofu cubes on a roasting tray. Roast in the oven for 15 minutes. Allow to cool. This stays tasty for a day or two when stored in an airtight container in the fridge.

Serves 3–4

TIP: I USUALLY MAKE THIS THE NIGHT BEFORE AND PACK IT FOR LUNCH THE NEXT DAY – THE FLAVOUR GETS BETTER OVERNIGHT!

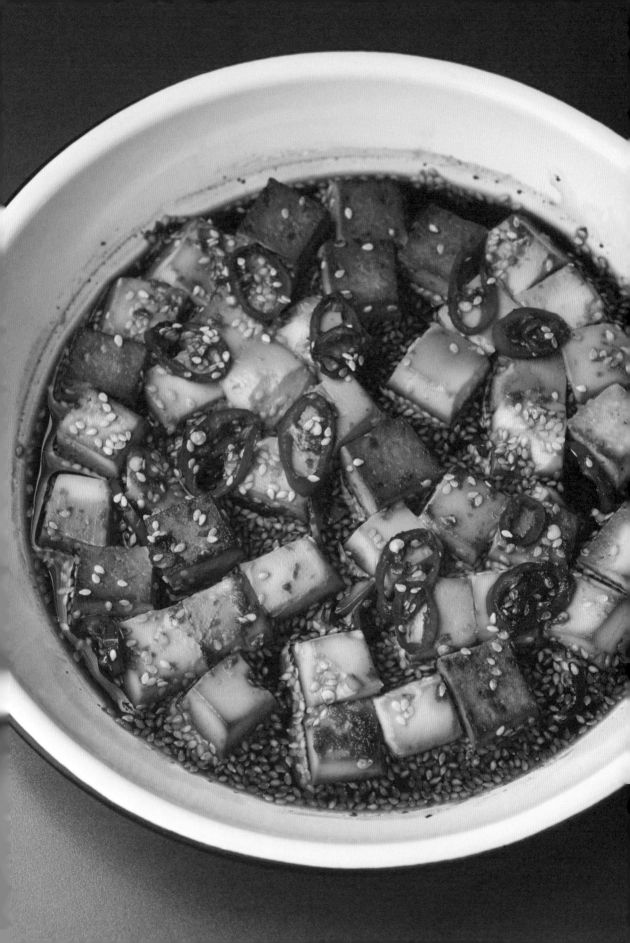

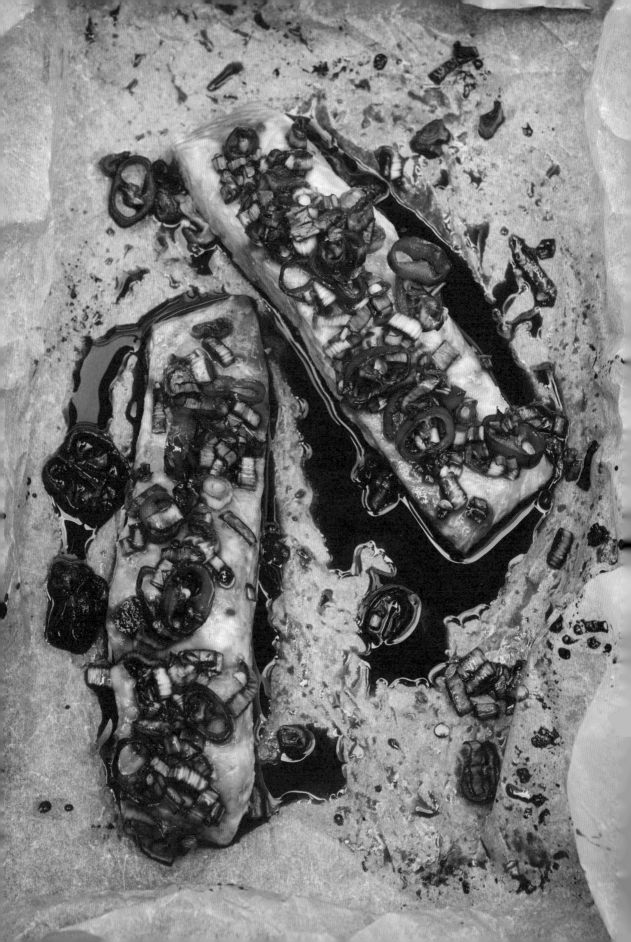

Roasted Glazed Salmon

This is requested at least once a week in our house.

Ingredients

2 tablespoons tamari

2 tablespoons honey

1 fresh chilli, finely chopped

3 spring onions, finely chopped

2 pieces salmon, skin on,
   approx. 150g each

Preheat the oven to 180°C.

To make the glaze, put the tamari, honey, chilli and spring onions in a small bowl, and mix to combine.

Place the salmon pieces on a baking tray, baste all over with glaze and place in the oven.

Every 3–5 minutes, baste the salmon with more glaze while it cooks. Bake for about 20 minutes or until cooked to your liking, and enjoy!

Serves 2

Alkalising Green Soup

Don't be frightened by how green this looks! Lauryn Eagle gave me this recipe when I was training (hard core) for the David Jones show and was trying to get as many greens into me as possible. I was so sceptical, even while I was making it. It's now my favourite soup!

Ingredients

1 tablespoon coconut oil

2 cloves garlic, peeled

2cm piece fresh ginger, peeled and grated

½ teaspoon ground coriander

½ teaspoon ground turmeric

pinch of pink sea salt

1 medium zucchini, roughly sliced into small pieces

500ml salt-reduced vegetable stock

½ cup broccoli, roughly chopped into small pieces

handful kale, finely chopped

juice of 1 lime

1 small bunch fresh parsley, roughly chopped

lime zest and fresh parsley, for garnish

Heat the oil in a wok or frying pan over medium heat, and add the garlic, ginger, coriander, turmeric and salt. Sauté over a low to medium heat for 2 minutes, then add 3 tablespoons of water. Add the zucchini, mixing well to coat the slices in all the spices, and cook for 3 minutes. Add 400ml of stock and simmer for a further 3 minutes. Add the broccoli, kale, lime juice and the rest of the stock. Cook for 3–4 minutes, or until all vegetables are soft.

Remove from the heat and add the chopped parsley. Pour everything into a blender and blend on a high speed until smooth. The soup will be a beautiful green with dark speckled bits of kale through it. Garnish with lime zest and parsley.

Serves 2

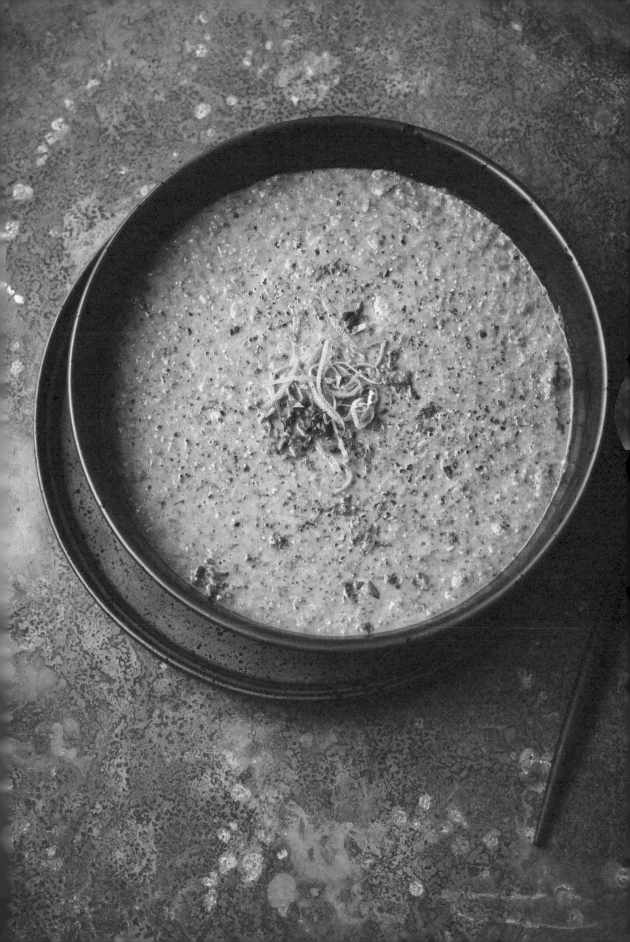

Chicken Stir-fry

This has been a dinner staple of mine since I moved out of home. I always take the leftovers to work for lunch.

Ingredients

2 chicken breast fillets, thinly sliced

1 tablespoon coconut oil

4 spring onions

½ long red chilli, deseeded

handful snow peas, trimmed

½ head broccoli, cut into bite-sized pieces

handful green beans, halved

¼ red cabbage, thinly sliced

handful baby spinach leaves

fresh basil leaves, for serving

cooked quinoa, for serving

Marinade

1 long red chilli, seeds included

3 cloves garlic, peeled and grated

2 tablespoons sesame oil

3 tablespoons tamari

Place all the marinade ingredients and the sliced chicken in a bowl. Marinate while preparing your veggies.

In a wok or large frying pan over medium heat, add the coconut oil, spring onions and fresh chilli. Sauté until the spring onions are cooked through. Remove the chicken from the marinade and reserve marinade. Add the chicken to the wok and cook halfway through then add the vegetables – this ensures the chicken is tender and not overcooked. Add the reserved marinade and cook until the vegetables are just tender and the chicken is cooked through.

Toss some fresh basil leaves through the stir-fry and serve with cooked quinoa.

Serves 2–4

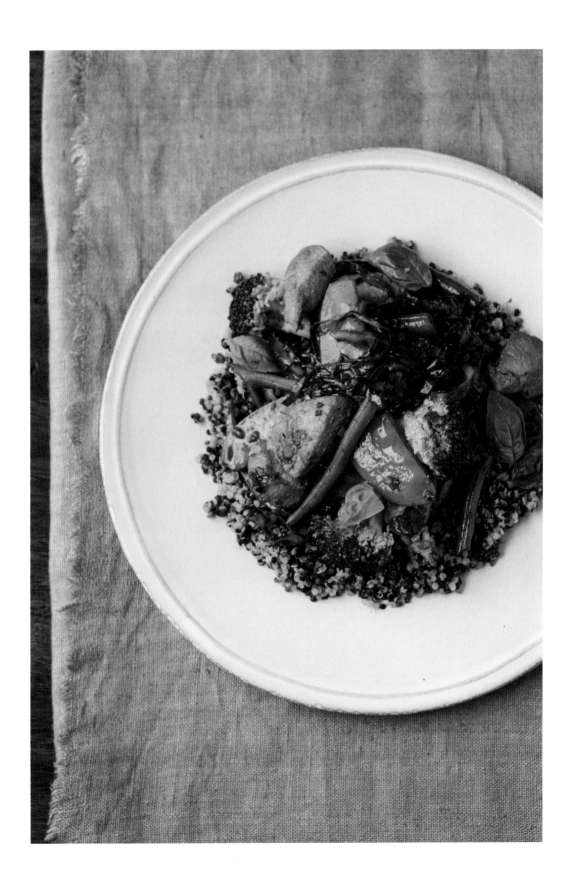

Zucchini Pasta with
Pesto

Dad makes an amazing penne pesto pasta. I replaced the penne with zucchini so I can still enjoy the meal with my family.

Ingredients

1 small bunch fresh basil

1 small bunch fresh coriander

1 long red chilli

4 cloves garlic, peeled

½ cup pine nuts

2 tablespoons coconut oil

1 large zucchini

salt and pepper

½ small bunch fresh parsley, chopped, for garnish

Wash the basil and remove the leaves (discarding the stalks). Wash the coriander – you're keeping the stalks for this so wash the roots thoroughly, there's usually a bit of grit there – and finely chop the chilli (keep the seeds in if you want extra spice). Place the basil, coriander, garlic and chilli into the bowl of your food processor with the pine nuts and the coconut oil. Pulse the mix until it's combined but not too chunky.

Trim off the ends of the zucchini and put through a spiralizer or make ribbons out of it with a vegetable peeler. You can either lightly fry the zucchini noodles in some coconut oil in a pan over a low heat for 2 minutes or bring a small pot of water to the boil and blanch them for a minute or two before draining. While the noodles are still hot, toss them in your pesto mixture before plating them. Season with salt and pepper and garnish with parsley. (This dish is delicious and the parsley might help with the garlic breath afterwards!)

Serves 1

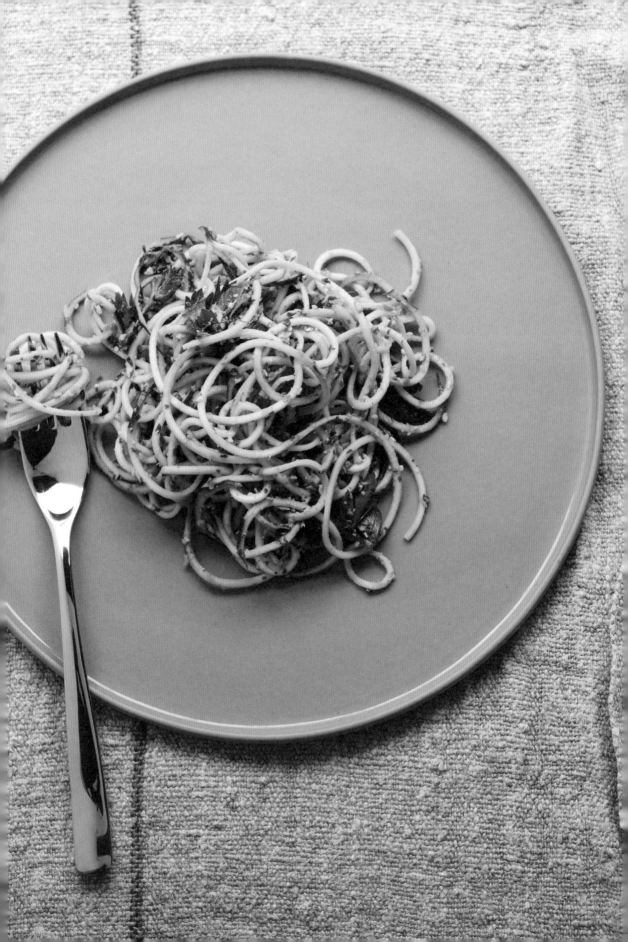

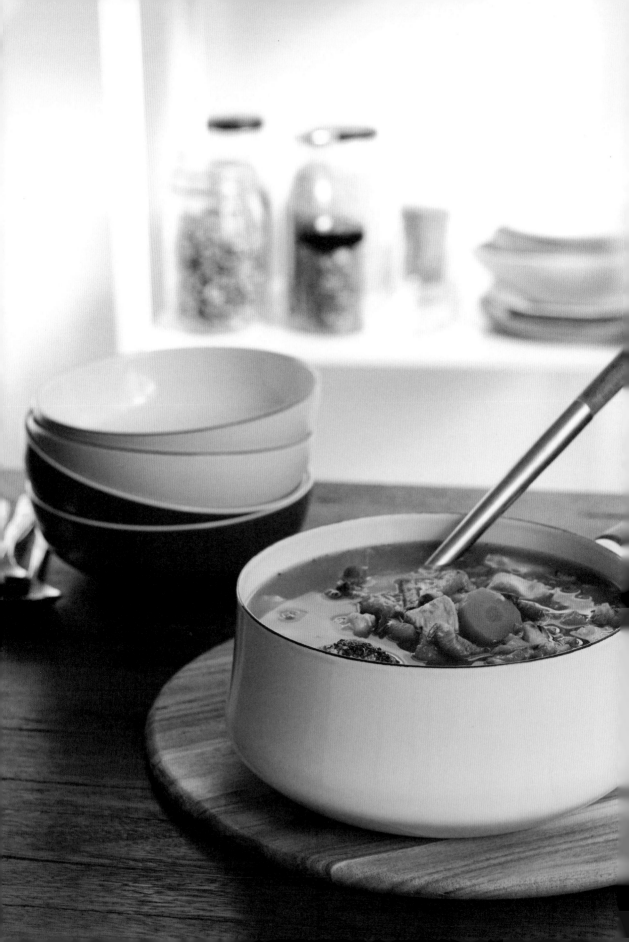

Chicken & Vegetable Soup

I've always been a fan of soup! Mum used to make epic pots of soup that we would continue to eat days later – the flavour just gets better every day.

Ingredients

4–5 cloves garlic, peeled and finely chopped

2 leeks, roughly chopped

2 large carrots, roughly chopped

1⅔ cups mushrooms (your choice, I like button or Swiss brown mushrooms for this recipe)

1 long red chilli, roughly chopped

1 tablespoon coconut oil

6–7 cups chicken broth (see page 132) or salt-reduced chicken stock

3 cups cold water

1 large sweet potato, peeled

2 chicken breasts approx. 300g total), skin removed

salt and pepper

1 medium head of broccoli

10–12 green beans, trimmed and halved

Place a large pot over low to medium heat and sweat the garlic, leeks, carrots, chilli and mushrooms with the coconut oil until they are soft. Add the chicken broth and 3 cups of cold water and allow the mix to gently simmer.

Chop the sweet potato into 2–3cm cubes and add to the simmering broth. Roughly chop the chicken breast into 2–3 cm cubes. Add to the broth and let the soup simmer over low to medium heat for 30–35 minutes. Skim off any foam that forms on the surface. Season with salt and pepper – taste to make sure it is to your liking.

Roughly chop the broccoli (use the stalks as well – they're delicious) and add to the soup with the beans, and let it simmer for a further 8 minutes. Turn off the heat and let the soup rest for a further 5 minutes before serving in large bowls.

You can freeze any leftover soup in an airtight container for up to a month.

Serves 4

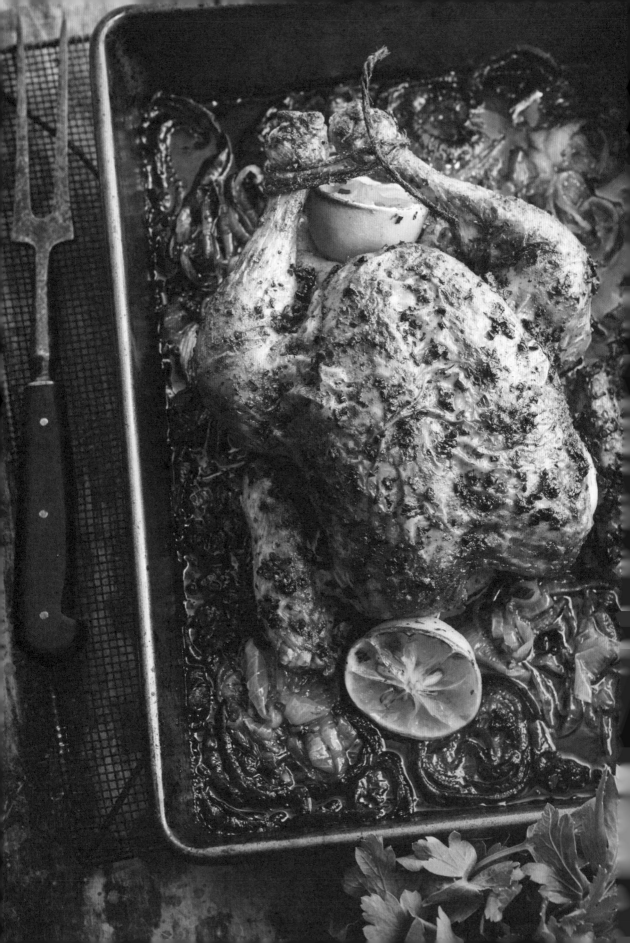

Roast Chicken

A Sunday fave of mine! I'm lucky if there is any left over.
If there is, I'll toss it through a salad or include it in an
omelette.

Ingredients

100g butter

3 cloves garlic, 2 peeled and
finely chopped, 1 for stuffing

1 long red chilli, finely sliced

zest of 1 lemon

1½ cups button mushrooms,
stalks trimmed

½ bunch parsley, finely chopped

pinch of pink sea salt

1 whole chicken, free range/
organic

½ lemon, for stuffing

Preheat the oven to 180°C.

In a small saucepan over medium heat, add
the butter, chopped garlic and chilli. When
the butter is melted, add the lemon zest,
mushrooms and parsley. Season with a pinch
of salt and cook until fragrant. Remove the pan
from the heat.

Separate the skin from the meat on the
chicken by carefully sliding a sharp knife
between the two. Carefully spoon the butter
and lemon mixture under the skin. Rub the
remaining mixture all over the skin on the
outside. Put the half lemon and extra clove of
garlic inside the chicken cavity.

Roast in the oven for approximately 1 hour
10 minutes (times will vary depending on the
size of the bird). Remove from the oven, cover
with foil and rest for 15 minutes before carving
and serving.

Serves 4

Turmeric Poached Chicken with
Brown Rice or Quinoa

Ingredients

½ cup brown rice or quinoa

2 medium skinless chicken breast fillets

4 cloves garlic, peeled and smashed

3cm piece fresh ginger, peeled and finely grated

2cm piece fresh turmeric, peeled and finely grated

2 bay leaves

1 teaspoon whole peppercorns

pinch of pink sea salt

½ small fresh red chilli (optional)

steamed bok choy, for serving (optional)

Place the brown rice in a small saucepan with 2–2½ cups water. Bring to a simmer over low to medium heat and cover. Leave gently bubbling for 35 minutes. All the water should be absorbed and the rice should be perfectly *al dente*. Check on it occasionally to make sure it isn't absorbing the water too quickly. If using quinoa, wash the grain thoroughly and drain, then cook according to the packet instructions.

While the rice or the quinoa is cooking, place the chicken fillets in a large saucepan. Add the garlic, ginger, turmeric, bay leaves, peppercorns and sea salt. Pour enough cold water over the ingredients to cover the fillets by about 2cm.

Place the saucepan over medium heat and bring the liquid to a boil then reduce the heat to a gentle simmer. You may like to skim any froth that forms as it simmers. The chicken should be cooked after about 10–14 minutes – check by removing one fillet and slicing into the middle to see if it is cooked through. When cooked, remove the chicken from the broth. Slice the poached chicken thinly and serve with the cooked quinoa or rice and optional steamed greens.

Serves 2

TIP: KEEP THE REMAINING POACHING LIQUID (FREEZES FOR A MONTH OR SO) TO USE IN THE SIMPLE CHICKEN BROTH (SEE PAGE 132).

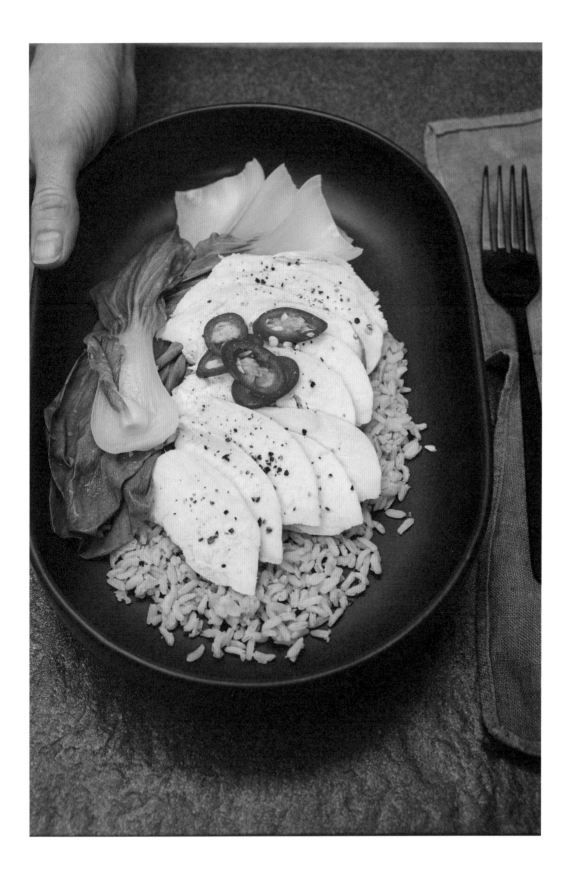

Honey-roasted Sweet Potato

Yum! Enough said.

Ingredients

1 tablespoon honey

2 tablespoons coconut oil

pinch of paprika

salt and pepper

1 sweet potato, peeled and
   chopped into chunks

Preheat the oven to 180°C.

Place the honey and coconut oil in a small saucepan over low heat. Once the honey and coconut oil have melted, stir to combine and add a pinch of paprika. Season with salt and pepper.

Place the sweet potato chunks into a roasting dish. Pour the honey mixture over the top, mix through evenly and roast until golden, usually about 25–30 minutes.

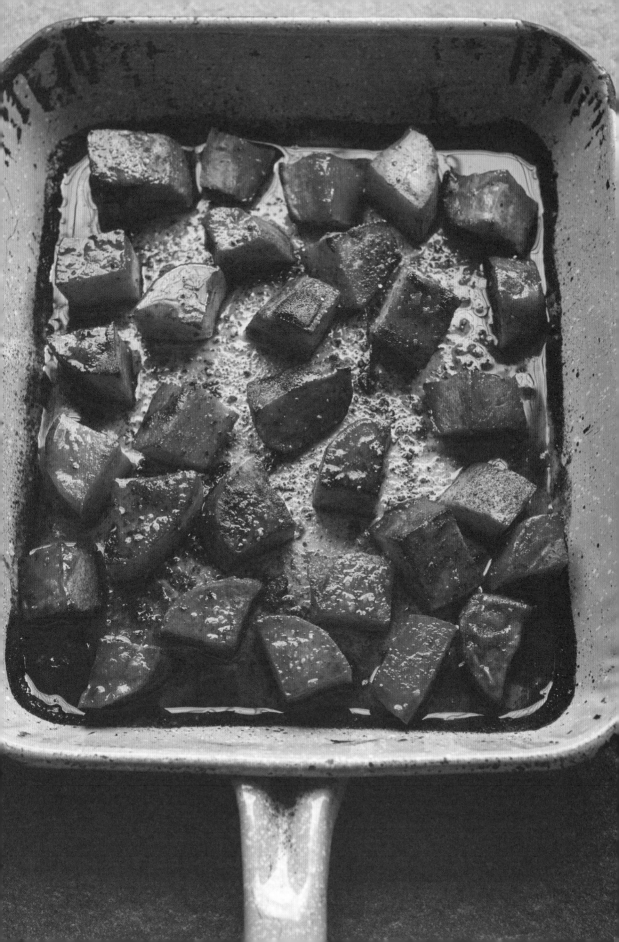

Steamed Greens with
Tamari and Toasted Sesame Seeds

Healthy, tasty and easy to make. This simple dish is the trifecta.

Ingredients

2 tablespoons sesame seeds

½ head broccoli, trimmed and cut into small florets

handful trimmed green beans

handful snow peas or sugar snap peas

½ tablespoon coconut oil

2 tablespoons tamari

Toast the sesame seeds in a wok until golden brown.

Steam all the greens over a boiling pot of water until the colour becomes vibrant. Remove immediately and set aside.

In a wok over medium heat, heat the coconut oil, add the greens and tamari and toss until combined. Remove from the heat. Sprinkle with the toasted sesame seeds and serve.

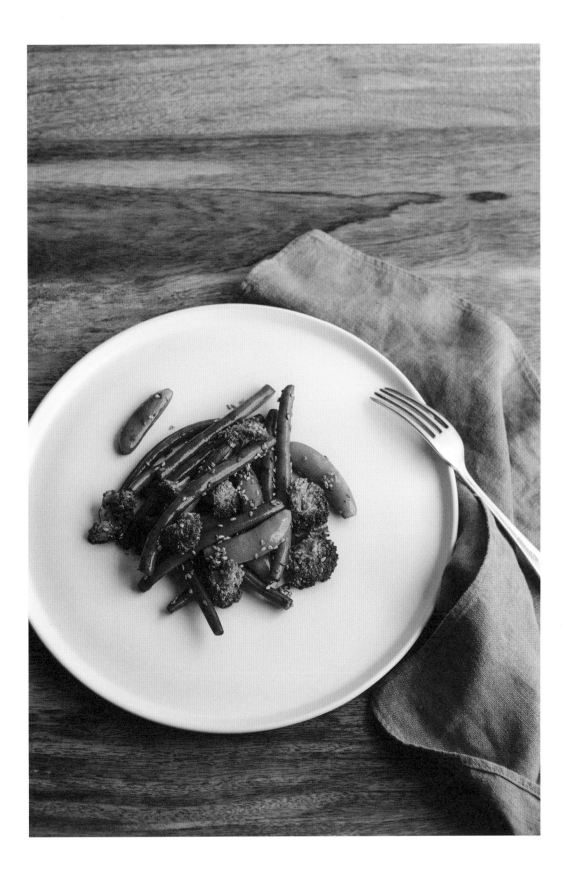

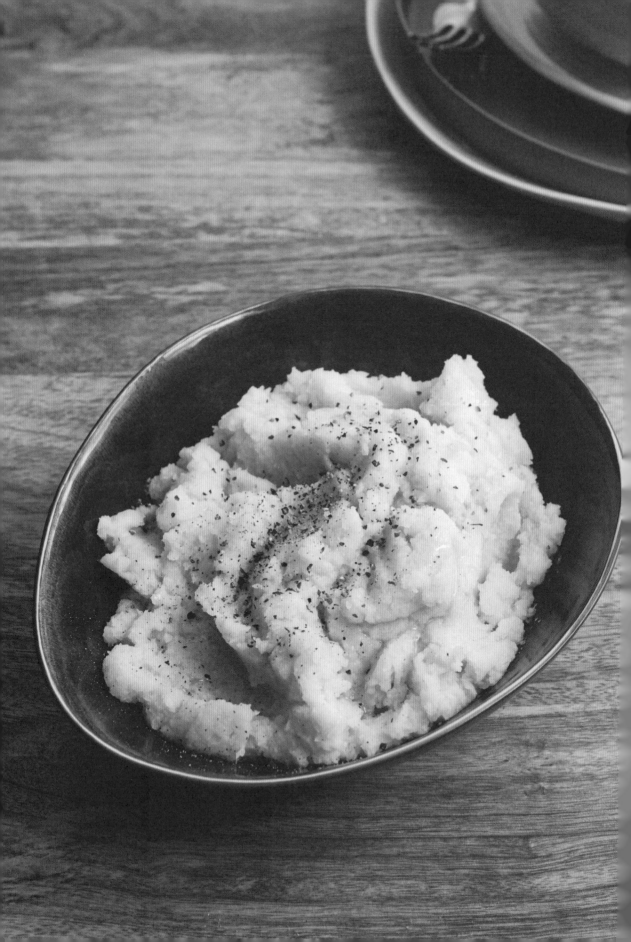

Cauliflower Mash

I adore mashed potato, and this is a healthier, lighter alternative. I once fooled a friend who declared she hated cauliflower. She was convinced it was mashed potato and even came back for seconds!

Ingredients

1 medium head of cauliflower, cut into small pieces

1 cup salt-reduced vegetable stock

1 teaspoon butter (optional)

cracked black pepper

Place the cauliflower and stock into a large saucepan over low to medium heat. Cover with a lid and simmer until the cauliflower is soft and cooked through.

Mash with a potato masher or blend in a processor until the cauliflower has a soft, smooth consistency. Add the butter if using, and combine until creamy. Season with lots of pepper.

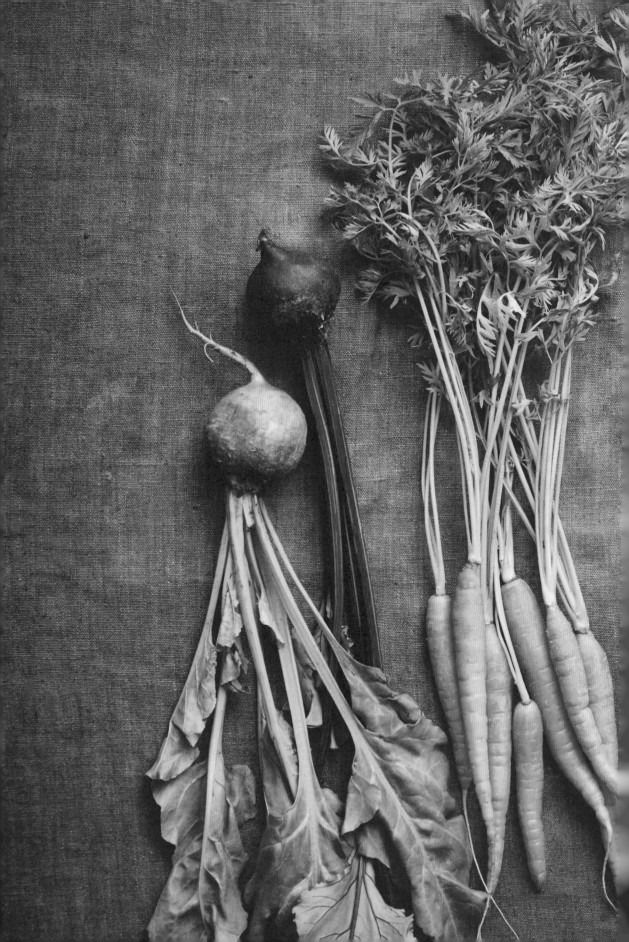

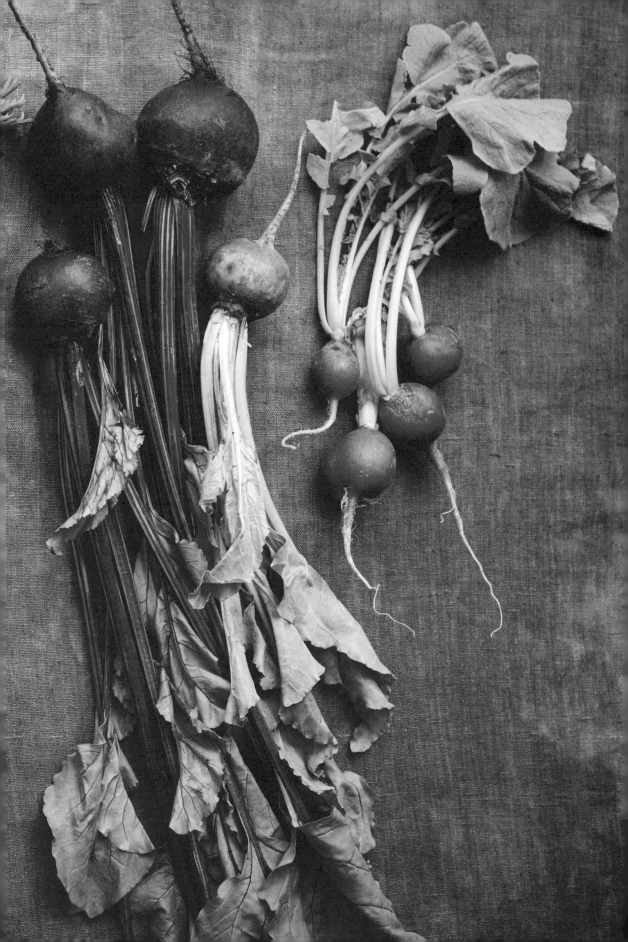

Big Dreams

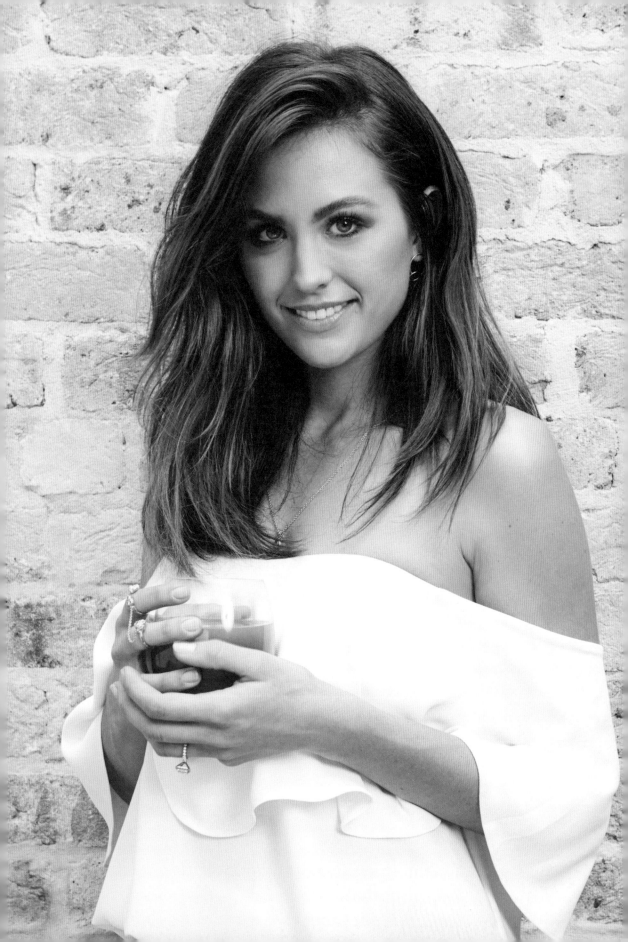

Let the journey begin

GROWING UP, I ALWAYS had a pretty good idea of what I wanted to do and what I had to do to get there, and I believe it's because I was introduced to goal setting from a young age.

When I was about fifteen, my mum took me through a modified version of something she had written for her employers to help them create a vision for their lives and careers. Every great person has a vision, so it only makes sense to create a vision for your life, something you stand by. Having a clear vision helps you to keep focused and whenever you're stuck making a decision or feeling a bit lost, you can refer back to your vision in order to seek clarity and set you on the right path.

My vision has nothing to do with career, success, money or anything materialistic. It's about who I want to be as a person and it is the statement behind most decisions I make in life. The same vision I wrote when I was fifteen is taped on the inside of my wardrobe where I can see it every day when I'm getting dressed. It's not something that I have shared publicly before; however, I wanted to share it with you in the hope that you can understand and feel inspired to write your own vision for your life.

My personal vision

'To help make the world brighter
by encouraging others to be the best person
they can be, by going after my dreams,
using my talents wisely and living
to my highest potential.'

As I sit here writing this book, I feel like I need to thank my fifteen-year-old self for writing down such a clear vision. I am doing what I am doing today because of this. There have been many ups and downs, but I can comfortably say that this is how I choose to live my life and every day when I have to make decisions I refer back to this vision and see whether or not it aligns. It has made business, career and life choices easier for me to make as I know what it is that I want to achieve; and if it doesn't sit within that vision, then I let it pass. It ensures that everything I do is genuine and authentic and I hope that shines through in everything you all get to see publicly.

I want to wish you all the best in setting your own vision. I have found it a very empowering tool in my life and business and I hope that you, too, have the same experience.

Before you begin I would like to leave you with my favourite quote, which was the final part of my speech as school captain on our graduating day and something I have always loved:

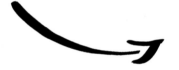

We ask ourselves,
WHO AM I TO BE
BRILLIANT, GORGEOUS,
TALENTED, FABULOUS?
Actually, who are
you not to be?

Your playing
small
does not
serve the
WORLD

- MARIANNE WILLIAMSON

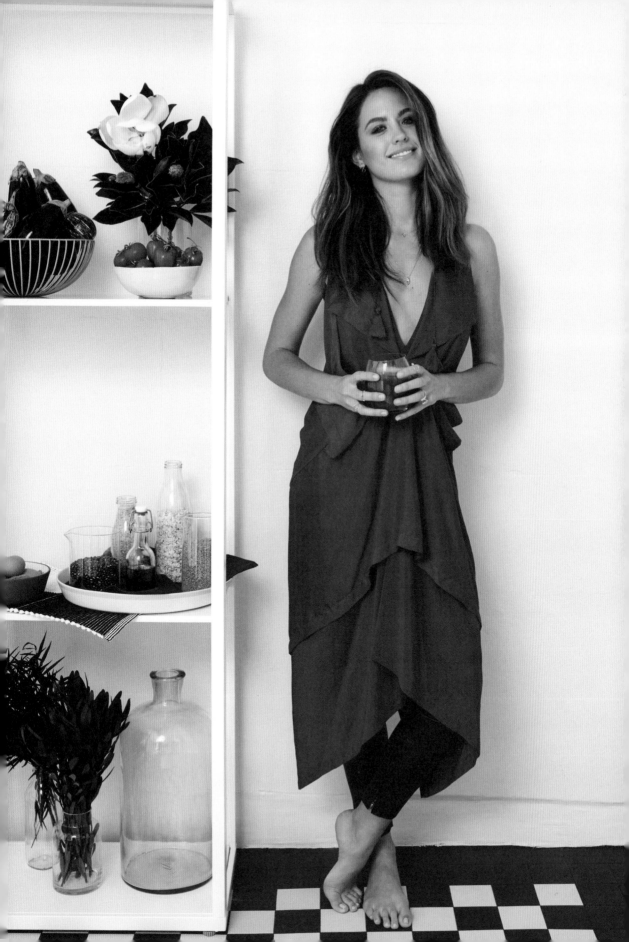

What's your vision?

IN DECIDING TO CREATE a personal vision statement, you are taking the first step to live your life by design rather than default.

So why would you do this?

A personal vision statement helps you express your purpose, your life's dream, what you want for yourself, and what you want to contribute to others. It engages your heart and spirit, gives you something to aim for, provides hope, gives meaning to the work you do and provides life direction. It helps you find your voice.

Without question, writing a vision statement can be one of the most powerful and significant things you can do to take leadership over your life. In writing it, you are taking a step to identify greater meaning in the work you do. It's like deciding which wall to lean your ladder of life against and then giving you a reason to climb. It will be a compass – a strong source of guidance amid any stormy seas and pulling currents in your life.

In a nutshell, a personal vision statement will create a framework for an empowering life, provide direction to guide the course of your days and help you make the best choices for yourself. It is your unique story for the world and gives expression to your life's journey.

Is that enough reason to invest your time?

So what does a vision statement look like?

Your vision is a simple statement of what you want to achieve in your life. Unlike a goal, it will change very little over time because it's big picture, always slightly out of reach so it pulls you along and becomes a guiding light in your life. It is grand and dreamy; however, it is kept grounded by ensuring it engages and gives expression to all of the following:

- Your talent – your gifts and strengths, i.e. those things that come naturally to you.

- Your passion – what you love to do in life, those things that energise, excite, motivate and inspire you.

- Your humanity – how you can make a difference to others or the world.

And to make it really fly, it's helpful if your statement meets a need in the world – that is, something you can be paid for. This makes your vision sit in a financially sustainable reality.

Finally, you write it down, and this anchors it to reality. That's why I keep my vision statement somewhere I can see it every day, so when I read it, it makes me feel excited, energised and creates a sense of fulfilment in knowing that it is my life vision – it inspires me into action!

Writing your vision statement

I am going to help by giving you a process, but first you need to understand it is not easy – although I can assure you it will be rewarding and worthwhile. It does require a commitment to yourself, a willingness to take a journey, to delve into your heart, mind and spirit to give expression to your life's vision.

However, once you have found it, there is no shortcut to living your vision. You will need to be prepared to grow, reflect on yourself, and push yourself to honour your responsibility for bringing your vision into reality. I promise you this – it will be the most challenging adventure you undertake. Be not afraid, as it will be in the challenges that you will find the pathway to living your dream.

So if you're ready, let's step up, step out and start the challenge today!

Be prepared to dig deep, go beneath the surface of your thoughts, to ask tough and engaging questions to uncover a real and empowered pathway to your legacy.

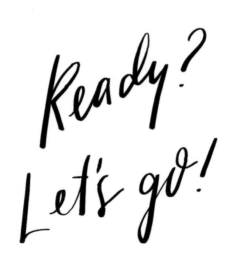

Your work journal

THIS PART OF THE book is to help guide and open your heart and mind to possibilities for your life. To explore your passions, talents and things that matter to you.

As you ponder the questions, your intentions should become clearer. Ideas and possibilities will open up.

If at any time working through this journal, you want to give up or your thoughts tell you it is a waste of time, push through by focusing on your completed personal vision in bright shining lights. These types of feelings are simply distractions and arise as a normal part of the change process. You can do it!

Visualisation

The first step on this journey is visualising your future self. Visualisation is a process that requires concentration and imagination. Find a quiet place where you can sit comfortably. Close your eyes and relax for a few minutes. Try not to think of anything in particular. When you feel calm, picture your ideal future – where you are, what job is fulfilling you, the people around you. Keep this image in your mind and focus on the details. Now expand outwards from the detailed points to view your possible future big picture!

From your future

From the visualisation, write down a list of words/statements that best describe your future self and environment.

Write down anything of significance for you that came out of the visualisation that you might want to reflect on at another time.

Write down any obvious changes to your present life you may want to make after seeing your future vision.

Where I am today

What are three things that are most meaningful to you in your life today?

1

2

3

Cast your mind back over the past few years of your life. What has been your main focus and where have you spent most of your time?

What sort of person have you been during that time?

If your life ended today, what would you regret not:

Doing

Seeing

Achieving

What are the things that you think you would be most remembered for?

Positive

Negative

What would these people say about you?

A friend from school or uni

Your best friend

Your partner

Your parents

Your siblings

A work mate

The recurring themes in my life have been:

Positive

Negative

My biggest challenges in life have been:

They have made me stronger by:

What I discovered about myself because of these challenges is:

The things I really enjoy doing are:

These issues/causes make me want to do something when I hear about them:

What are the five most important values in my life? (Circle)

Having integrity

Being fit and healthy

Having a nice home and belongings

Leaving the world a better place

Having fun

Being honest

Learning and improving myself

Making others' lives easier or more pleasant

Enjoying/supporting my family

My spirituality or religion

Others (write down what they are)

These are the things I can do at the good-to-excellent level:

Three things I'd do if I won lotto tomorrow:

1

2

3

What are the things I'd like to stop doing or do as little as possible? (Be specific – don't just say 'work', say what it is about the work that you want to stop.)

_____

_____

I found these things easy to do as a child:

_____

_____

What strengths have other people commented on about me and my accomplishments?

_____

_____

The main things that motivate me or bring me joy and satisfaction are:

_____

Four of my greatest strengths/abilities/traits/things I do best are:

1	
2	
3	
4	

What are the ten things I most enjoy doing? (Be honest. These are the ten things without which your life would feel incomplete.)

1	
2	
3	
4	
5	
6	
7	
8	
9	
10	

What three things in your work . . .

	Do you love	Do you dislike	Would give you a greater sense of fulfilment
1			
2			
3			

Write your perfect job description.

What are the things that you most often search for on the internet or social media?

If you were to enrol in a course tomorrow, purely for pleasure, what would you study?

What are the specific skills, knowledge and talents that are unique gifts you can share with others?

Time for the big questions about the world

What ignites your passion? Circle those that spark your interest:

Administration	Agriculture	Animal Care	Animal Protection
Animal Rights	Art	Books	Broadcasting
Business	Caring for the elderly	Child Care	Child Protection
Children	Civil Rights Issues	Community Development	Construction
Creativity	Defence	Design	Education
Energy	Entertainment	Environment	Family Issues
Fashion	Finance	Food	Gardening
Government	Health Care	Homelessness	Human Development
Illness & Disability	Immigration	Infants	Journalism
Justice	Law	Literacy	Management
Media	Mental Health	Movies	Music
News	Non-Profit Agencies	Nursing	Nutrition
Parks & Recreation	Performing Arts	Politics	Poverty
Printing & Publishing	Psychology	Public Safety	Real Estate
Rehabilitation	Religion	Reproductive Issues	Research
Science	Sexuality Issues	Space Exploration	Spirituality
Sports	Teaching	Technology	Tourism
Travel	Veterans	Women's Issues	Youth

What do you dream about; what holds you spellbound?

Whose work or life inspires you?

What are you doing when you feel inspired?

What would you talk about if given an hour of prime time TV to influence the nation or the world?

If you were to start an organisation tomorrow to solve a world need, what would it be?

What are three things you would do if you knew you could not fail?

1

2

3

How would you use a gift of ten million dollars if it had to be given away to a cause, issue or problem that moves you?

What I most want to be remembered for is:

_____

What I most want out of life is:

_____

The exploring is done – time to craft your personal vision statement

You are ready now to create the masterpiece . . . your story.

Remember, a vision statement is an expression of how you will manifest your legacy. It is the fulfilment of your unique gifts and passion and speaks powerfully about the person you are and the person you are becoming. It is written to inspire you, guide you and give expression to your story – it is for you.

Sample vision statements to help

Here are a few ideas to get you started:

- To promote and advocate high quality care to the critically ill and injured so that people's lives can be enhanced. I will do this by teaching, encouraging and supporting healers.

- To put an end to animal abuse by educating the world about the joy that animals can bring to a person's life and how they can improve the quality of life.

- To promote and encourage cultural diversity in order to help disadvantaged children live in safety.

- To enrich the human experience by reducing suffering for families in times of sickness by lending a helping hand.

- To bring joy and love into the world through an appreciation of animals by volunteering.

- To enable children to live in a loving, healthy and safe environment by raising parenting awareness and skill.

- To support children to grow and become healthy, happy adults through creating and offering learning programs that enhance wellbeing.

- To create homes that people love to live in and enhance wellbeing.

- To provide gardens that bring joy and happiness to people who walk in them.

- To use my strengths to support others to see their potential and step up to take responsibility for leading an extraordinary life.

The steps

Aim for around 50 words or less – however, it is better to fully articulate the vision you want for your life and your future, than be limited by word count, so do what you need to do to express your vision clearly.

1. Read over and reflect on what you have written so far in the work journal.

2. Reflecting on your answers will help you to build a bank of words that you really like, inspire you and that you could use to help write your vision. Below is a list to help you; circle the ones you like and add in your own:

create	develop	enthuse	enable
empower	generate	guide	model
support	greatness	inspire	aspire
become	build	think	grow
care	promote	believe	nurture
share	play	expand	provide
accomplish	dedicate	commit	resilience
imagine	enrich	advocate	

3. Now use the space on the next page to help draft a statement. You will need to write more than one draft so keep going with it until you feel happy.

I will . . . (what you want to achieve, do or become)

_____

_____

4. Taking the draft statement, wordsmith it and work to tighten up and shorten the statement until you feel it accurately reflects a vision for you. It can be helpful to find someone to work with if you need assistance at this stage.

--- --- --- --- --- --- --- --- --- --- --- --- --- --- --- --- --- ---

TIP: YOU WILL KNOW YOU ARE CLOSE WHEN YOU FEEL A CONNECTION TO THE WORDS AND ARE EXCITED ABOUT THEM. YOU ARE LOOKING FOR A BROAD-REACHING STATEMENT THAT WILL MAKE YOU FEEL PASSIONATE ABOUT YOUR LIFE EVERY TIME YOU READ IT.

--- --- --- --- --- --- --- --- --- --- --- --- --- --- --- --- --- ---

5. Once you have something you feel happy with, share it with a friend and ask them to challenge you about it so that you can further enhance it.

6. Finally, take your vision statement and create a visual masterpiece for you to put up somewhere you can see it every day and start sharing it with the world, whether that's at your desk or at home.

My vision statement is . . .

Living and sharing your dream

WELL DONE! IT IS quite a journey of exploration you have been on and you have arrived at the goal of your personal vision.

However, this is not the end of the story, it is just the beginning. Keep in mind that your personal vision statement can and will change over time, depending upon what is happening in your life. You will be amazed, however, at how many components do remain consistent over time. Every year, challenge and refine your statement; life evolves, and so will your vision.

Have the courage to talk about your vision and share it with others. It is in the sharing that you find the connections needed with others to create your dream. Humanity is one long connected chain – sharing and having conversations helps to bring everyone closer together.

And my final tip for success – work your dream

Connect with a fellow vision traveller and every week check in and commit to creating one small, specific and do-able action to move toward your vision. Take the KISS – Keep It Small and Simple – approach: a weekly KISS for your vision should not be too hard to remember 😄 and you will succeed.

Make it an action that will not take long, is easy to achieve and is going to keep you moving forward. This will give you a total of 52 forward actions every year . . . WOW! You will succeed in keeping your vision living and growing with this approach.

All the best with your journey –

I have NO doubt it will be amazing!

Index

Index

Acknowledgements

WOW! I ACTUALLY CANNOT believe that I am sitting down to write a page of 'Acknowledgements' for a book – I mean, my book!

I say it's my book but it wouldn't have even looked like a book if it wasn't for a team of beautiful, kind, genuine, funny people who made it all possible.

Firstly, to Robert, I don't just want to thank you for the copious amount of matcha green tea you made us for every catch up we had to discuss the book (it was a lot of tea!), I also want to thank you for guiding me through this entire process. I was so nervous about creating this book, but your encouragement the entire way through has made this experience something I will never forget. I still want to hang out and drink matcha tea even after it's all done – you're stuck with me now! And of course I couldn't thank Robert without thanking Murray – sorry we took over your kitchen for three weeks; you're the best ever, we love you and Robert and I owe you an awesome Christmas present!

As mentioned above, this creation really was a team effort and I was truly blessed to have the beautiful Patricia 'Patsy' Niven fly in from the UK to shoot all of the images for the book. We had never met before but as soon as we were introduced I felt like I had known her for years. Her warmth and infectious positivity made my days shooting with her so enjoyable. We shared many a laugh and every time I look through the book I'll think of Patsy.

Jeremy, aka 'Jez', thank you for your patience and for keeping us all on track. You put up with our nonsense all too nicely; you were an amazing part of our team!

Astred, the master book designer. There is not a single detail you have overlooked; you have given this book the personality and character we wanted. You have done an incredible job, thank you for being so talented!

Vikki and Sian, the food styling was NEXT LEVEL! You achieved everything I wanted and more. You brought the vision I had for the food presentation to life. I am so lucky to have had you both work on my book, I can't stop looking at the pictures of the food and produce. Incredible.

Liz, can you move in with me permanently!? Please? You had such a big job and I could not be happier with how it all turned out, thank you.

Aleysha, Normie and Max. Thank you all so much for everything. I am so fortunate that I get to work with you not only on this shoot but all the time on various jobs. All three of you are absolute heaven and never fail to brighten my day and this book shoot was no different.

I'd like to give a special mention to my Aunty Cynthia. From a young age you inspired me to think differently about food. I have so many wonderful memories of you in the kitchen and of our families all sitting around the table enjoying good food. You have taught me and inspired me more than you know, I am so grateful.

Thanks and acknowledgement must also go to my one of a kind, honest and inspiring mum. When you sat me down as a teenager and helped me write a vision and mission statement, little did I know it would lead to so many wonderful things, but deep down I think you always knew. Mum and Dad, this book is a (very) small display of the wisdom and guidance you have given me.

Finally, my best friend and soul mate. Thank you for not complaining once when the computer was set up in the lounge room for months on end as I typed away while you watched TV. I owe you one hundred cuddles for every time you went to bed and I stayed up working on this. X

IMPORTANT NOTE TO READERS: Although every effort has been made to ensure the contents of this book are accurate, it must not be treated as a substitute for qualified medical advice. Always consult a qualified medical practitioner. Neither the author nor the publisher can be held responsible for any loss or claim arising out of the use, or misuse, of the suggestions made or the failure to take professional medical advice.

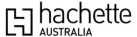 **hachette**
AUSTRALIA

Published in Australia and New Zealand in 2016
by Hachette Australia
(an imprint of Hachette Australia Pty Limited)
Level 17, 207 Kent Street, Sydney NSW 2000
www.hachette.com.au

10 9 8 7 6 5 4 3 2 1

National Library of Australia
Cataloguing-in-Publication data:

Campbell, Jesinta, author.
Live a beautiful life / Jesinta Campbell.

978 0 7336 3570 0 (paperback)

Campbell, Jesinta.
     Celebrities – Australia – Biography.
     Cooking.
     Health.
     Beauty, Personal.
     Self-actualization (Psychology) in women.

791.45092

Cover and text design by Astred Hicks, Design Cherry
Photography by Patricia Niven
Photography Assistants: Jeremy Wolf, David Rex
Hair and makeup by Norman Gonzales and Max May
Home Economy by Elizabeth Chapman
Styling by Sian Redgrave
Styling by Vikki Moursellas

Thanks to David Jones for providing props for styling.

Colour reproduction by Splitting Image
Printed in China by Toppan Leefung